MEAL PREPPING FOR WOMEN'S WEIGHT LOSS

MEAL-PREP PLANS AND RECIPES ADAPTABLE
TO YOUR FAMILY AND YOUR WEIGHT-LOSS
PROGRAM

ROBYN BROOKS

Dedicated to my dear Wade and Cassey who have supported me every step of my journey back to health. Your love means the world to me.

Dear Reader,

The meal planners will help you stay focused throughout the week, which will help you reach your goals. You may make copies of the planners if you would like.

If you would like the planners included in printable form, please scan the QR code below, or send an email to:

brooksmealprepbooks@gmail.com

I hope you enjoy this book and find it extremely valuable on your meal prep and weight loss journey.

Please take a couple of minutes to leave a review on Amazon when you have a moment.

Thank you,
Robyn Brooks

CONTENTS

INTRODUCTION

Most women have at some point grappled with weight-related issues, be it weight loss, weight gain, or weight maintenance. All these issues are to some extent food related. Many of us know the importance of diet and the impact of food on our bodies, so it's not for lack of knowledge that we are faced with these challenges but rather due to lack of time. We lead such busy lives juggling work, school, family, friends, and so forth that thinking about what we eat tends to fall by the wayside. Planning and preparing meals in advance is the best way to ensure we eat healthily to achieve our weight goals—weight-loss goals in particular—and minimize the stress that comes with trying to figure out what to prepare for dinner every day and grabbing what's available for lunch just to get rid of the hunger pangs.

Through my own weight-loss journey, I learned that the key to successful weight loss is planning and preparing meals on a weekly basis. By doing this, I was able to make healthy choices and remove the possibility of grabbing a bag of chips because I was too tired to cook.

The aim of this book is to teach you hassle-free ways of meal prepping and planning that will get a meal on your table in a short time.

You can choose any meal-prep plan in the book, or you can start with the simplest—planning and prepping for one meal a week—and work your way to meal prepping and planning for a month at a time. This book will assist you in streamlining meal preparation and getting out of the kitchen quickly. You will learn how to plan, cook, and alter meals to meet the specific demands of your family and personal circumstances. This book will help you

- take the guesswork out of meal prepping
- know how to store your meals properly
- create a seamless meal prep process

By the end of this book, you will be able to comfortably adapt any of the meal-prep plans shared with you to your lifestyle and schedule.

The information in this book is meant to empower you with information, encourage you to take control of your eating, and help you make healthier food choices.

1

IS IT REALLY HARDER FOR WOMEN TO LOSE WEIGHT?

It's a fact—men lose weight faster than women. Several studies have been carried out through the years to determine if there are differences in how men and women lose weight.

The Research

When 11 studies were analyzed, 10 of them found that men lost significantly more weight in kilograms, more body fat, and a higher percentage of belly fat than women.

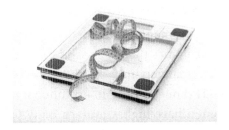

This was also documented in the journal *Diabetes, Obesity and Metabolism* in August 2018 (Christensen et al., 2018). For the study, over 2,000 overweight, prediabetic men and women were monitored by researchers over 8 weeks as they followed an 800-calorie diet.

Let's take a moment to talk about calories. Most of us associate calories with how fattening a food is. In fact, though, calories relate to the quantity of energy that a food delivers in terms of nutrition. We gain weight if we consume more energy than we require on a regular basis. However, we will lose weight and fat if we consume insufficient energy.

Body Composition

Because of their body composition, men tend to have a higher metabolic rate and more muscle mass than women. Men have more visceral fat in their midsection, and when people lose fat in their midsection, they burn more fat because their metabolic rate increases. According to research, fat cells in the abdomen are more sensitive and release fat more easily than fat cells in the hips and thighs. Men burn approximately 400 calories per day more than women.

Conversely, women carry more fat in the hip, thigh, and rear areas. This is called subcutaneous fat, and the loss of this fat has been shown to have no impact on the metabolic rate and the fat-burning process.

Hormones

Because of estrogen, women are inclined to carry between 6% and 11% more fat in their bodies than men, and their lower muscle mass makes weight-loss maintenance harder for women. Women's increased body fat is thought to be an evolutionary adaptation to aid in pregnancy. Women have higher average body fat than men from puberty to menopause despite consuming fewer calories. However, it is critical to remember that 'fat' in this case does not imply 'unhealthy.' Yes, women have more fat stores than men, but this is part of their physiology, so it's not just extra weight. Women should have 20%–25% body fat while men should have 10%–15%. Men and women are different even at healthy body fat levels, so just because a woman has 11% more body fat than a man doesn't mean she's 11% 'fatter.' A woman who is perfectly fit will still have a higher body fat percentage than a man who is perfectly fit—about 6%–11% more. Furthermore, men tend to lose weight where they need to lose it the most—their bellies—so it is often more noticeable when men begin to trim down than when women do. Women's fat stores are typically more dispersed, which is partly why their weight-loss rate is slower than that of men. Simple, regular exercise of 30–60 minutes daily has been shown to shift abdominal fat, even if overall weight is not reduced. So, while women may lose abdominal fat as quickly as men; they just have less of it.

Nutritional Requirements

When it comes to nutrition, the required protein, carbohydrate, and fat breakdowns are the same for both men and women, but men require more calories and a larger overall consumption of each macronutrient. Women require fewer calories than men, but they frequently require more vitamins and minerals. Women generally need more folic acid, calcium, and iron. Consuming the right amounts of nutrients is a critical component of weight loss. So, if a woman is eating the same foods as a man, but she is not getting the correct nutrients, her weight loss will likely be slower.

Women are prone to weaker bones and osteoporosis than men due to hormonal changes linked with childbearing and menstruation. As a result, a postmenopausal woman requires more calcium than a man in the same age group (1,000 mg for 51- to 70-year-old women compared to 800 mg for 51- to 70-year-old men). At other ages, calcium consumption recommendations are the same for both genders. Over and above that, women often experience bouts of stress eating as a result of hormonal fluctuations associated with the menstrual cycle. The menstrual cycle is unique to women and is the primary reason for iron-deficient anemia being more prevalent in women than in men. The average premenopausal woman needs around 18 mg of iron per day, whereas men require just 8 mg. It's important to keep this, and all nutrients, in mind when creating an eating plan.

Metabolic Syndrome

Women are also more likely to suffer from metabolic syndrome than men. Organizations such as the World Health Organization, the American Association of Clinical Endocrinologists, the European Group for Study of Insulin Resistance, the American Heart Association, the International Diabetes Foundation, and the National Heart, Lung, and Blood Institute (NHLBI) all have their own criteria in terms of the requirements for a metabolic syndrome diagnosis, but what they all agree on is what it constitutes. Metabolic syndrome is a combination of hypertension, obesity, and diabetes. Each of these conditions is harmful to the body and overall health on its own, but a combination of all three can be deadly. The NHLBI states that a metabolic syndrome diagnosis will be made if at least three of the following are evident:

- raised body mass index (BMI)
- low high-density lipoprotein (HDL) cholesterol (in women, this would be below 50 mg/dL; in men, this would be below 40 mg/dL)
- a waist circumference of 35 inches for women and 40 inches for men
- hypertension, which would be a blood pressure of 130 mm Hg or higher systolic (the top number) or 85 mm Hg diastolic (the bottom number), or blood pressure medication has already been prescribed
- a triglyceride level of 150 mg/dL or above (triglycerides are a type of fat found in the blood)

Hypoglycemia is a considerably larger factor to the metabolic syndrome in women, whereas hypertension and elevated triglycerides are significantly larger contributors to the metabolic syndrome in men. This indicates that a healthy diet with a focus on blood sugar regulation could help reduce the risk of metabolic syndrome in women.

In both genders, the contribution of the various metabolic components to the metabolic syndrome differs. This could play a role in disparities in the relative risk of metabolic problems, like insulin resistance, between men and women. Studies also show that while the risk of developing metabolic syndrome increases with age in both genders, men are only four times more likely to develop metabolic syndrome as they age while women are six times more likely to develop it as they age.

Additional Research

According to research, there is also a link between socioeconomic disparities and metabolic syndrome in White, Black, and Mexican American women, but not in men.

Another interesting fact to note is that because excess fat is part of women's physiological makeup, women can gain weight even if they follow healthier eating habits or exercise regularly. Most men gain weight as a result of a high-calorie diet and a lack of physical activity combined. For most women, researchers found that it only takes one of these factors to cause weight gain.

Research also indicates there are differences in the foods that men and women prefer. Women are more likely to consume dairy products and foods high in added sugars, whereas men consume more meat-based foods. Furthermore, women are more likely than men to cope with stress through food. Emotional eating can be caused by low self-esteem, depression, or cultural or social factors that influence food choices and eating habits. NO evidence is needed to determine that eating high calorie foods while stressed can contribute to a woman's weight gain.

Much of the research indicates that yes, it can be more difficult for a woman to lose weight. Therefore, women must be diligent in planning what foods they eat. Maintaining a healthy weight is the most effective strategy to treat and prevent metabolic syndrome or overweight in general, and following a healthy diet that is low in sugar and fats and high in vegetables and fruit is an important part of achieving that.

2

HOW MEAL PREPPING CAN HELP WITH WEIGHT LOSS

We eat in our homes, at work, in restaurants, and maybe even in our cars. In some of these places, we have more control over what choices are available than in others. Also, picture this scenario: You left work late, your stomach is rumbling, and you have neither the energy nor the inclination to shop and cook. Your first stop? Takeout.

One of the main reasons people choose quick takeout meals, which are often high in calories and contribute to weight gain, is that their schedule is so busy. Since high-calorie foods are everywhere, it's important to take the time to plan ahead to make sure you have healthy options available.

Now picture a different scenario: You get home and you have a delicious home-cooked dinner, possibly even lunch packed for the next day, within a few minutes of walking through the door. In the midst of hectic weekday schedules, advance meal prep is a great tool to help us stay on track with our eating habits. Although all types of meal preparation necessitate planning, there is no one correct method, and it varies depending on food preferences, cooking ability, schedules, and personal goals.

Whether you're cooking for just yourself, for two, or for more people, preparing meals ahead is a good starting place when it comes to improving your food choices. Women may have to work harder to lose weight no matter what weight-loss program they use, but planning ahead can make it easier. Meal prepping allows you to choose optimal ingredients, rotate food options, and plan portion sizes, which are possibly the most important factors in achieving your weight-loss goals. A web-based observational NutriNet-Santé study polled 40,554 participants, and a total of 57% of those polled stated that they plan meals on a regular basis. Meal planners had a greater rate of adhering to nutrition guidelines and a decreased risk of becoming overweight.

One Kaiser-Permanente weight-loss study found that participants who kept a food journal lost about two times the weight of those who did not. Writing down what you will eat each week on a meal planning sheet is essentially a food journal, and could work for you the way it worked for the people in the study. Additionally, comparing the planning sheets with your hunger, weight gain or loss, join pain, and other physical measurements will bring to light things like over-consumption of food, hunger triggers, inflammatory triggers, and the likes. This form of journaling will make meal prepping more relevant, and you be more apt to find what really works for you on an individual basis.

Researchers in a Nutrition Research and Practice study have also found that rotating foods helps with weight loss. In the study, they were able to correlate food rotations helped with reducing abdominal fat, lowering HDL-cholesterol levels, and led to better fasting blood sugar levels. The researchers concluded that rotating healthy foods could prevent metabolic syndrome.

Still, another study published in the journal Advanced Nutrition found that eating a variety of colorful foods was linked to lower incidence of heart disease and obesity. Planning to eat vegetables and preparing those vegetables ahead of time is just one way meal prepping can improve your eating and help you reach those weight loss goals.

Benefits of Meal Prepping

The benefits of meal prepping are many, and some of them are outlined below:

Saves time

The truth is, for many of us there just aren't enough hours in a day, so meal planning removes at least one thing from our daily to-do list. When you first start meal planning, try to identify one meal where you really need a time saver or you really need to eat healthier, and then plan your prepping around that meal. Save time and eat healthy on your busiest days by having meals ready to go or by planning simple, quick meals that the whole family will enjoy. Finding the time to eat healthier can help with weight loss goals.

Lessens stress

Do you want to know what the biggest benefit of meal prepping is for me? Not having to worry about what's for dinner on my way home from work. Trying to figure out what's for dinner can be stressful, and planning and preparing meals in advance helps reduce the stress, especially on weeknights. Before meal prepping, I would even cause myself stress if I grabbed something unhealthy on my way home from work. Guilt about weight gain can be stressful, and stress has been shown to contribute to weight gain.

Ensures more control over what is eaten

Meal planning is associated with increased food variety, which is an important component of a healthy diet because it increases the likelihood of meeting nutrient needs and makes healthy eating less boring. More importantly, cooking at home gives you control and choice over the ingredients. Avoiding problematic food allergens and incorporating ingredients that support diets for your specific health are easier to manage. Controlling what you eat is the most important component of any weight loss program, and meal prepping makes this easier.

Uses less energy

It isn't uncommon for most of us to go grocery shopping two or more times per week—either we forget something, or we don't buy enough on the first trip to last a week. Meal planning streamlines your shopping because you make your grocery list based on your meal-prep plan—this ensures you get everything you need in a single trip. Not only does this cut down on the time spent at the grocery store, but it also saves you the costs in time and gas of making back-and forth-trips to the store. Let's face it, too often when we go to the grocery store, we end up buying tempting foods; why not limit those temptations to support your weight loss?

Makes health goals easier to achieve

Home-cooked meals tend to be lower in calories than takeout meals. They also have lower levels of sugar and sodium and more vegetables, which translates to more fiber and fewer saturated fats and carbohydrates. But not all vegetables and fruits are created equal—some may not be ideal for weight loss because of their nutrient composition. More on this a bit later.

Studies show that as the number of weekly meals prepared at home increases, so does the overall diet quality, helping lower the risk of developing type 2 diabetes. Cooking meals at home increases your chances of meeting health goals, whether they are to lose weight, improve heart health, or maintain blood sugar control. Meal planning is essential to achieve this.

When meal planning, including some foods from each food group is critical. Foods chosen from only one food group are neither nutritionally balanced nor appealing; for example, a chicken cooked with lentils in yogurt will be high in protein but low in minerals and vitamins due to the absence of vegetables.

Variety in your meals is very important because it ensures you get all the nutrients you need and at the same time helps prevent the boredom of eating the same foods frequently. So, incorporate a variety of fruits and vegetables, keeping in mind, as mentioned earlier, that some fruits and vegetables might not be ideal for helping you lose or maintain weight.

According to research, it is possible that high-glycemic-index carbohydrates are triggers for food addiction. Further research has demonstrated that the higher the glycemic load of a food, the more the body craves even more food. When deciding on what to eat, opt for foods in the low-glycemic index and low-glycemic load categories over those in the high-glycemic categories, save those in the middle for a special treat, and avoid those in the high range. All the sample plans and recipes in this book are created using these principles and can easily be adapted to what your family needs or prefers by adding oils, cheeses, or starches.

The glycemic index is easy to figure out:

- **Low glycemic index (GI 55 or below):** Most fruits and vegetables, low-fat dairy foods, beans, and nuts have a low glycemic index.
- **Moderate glycemic index (GI 56 to 69):** Corn, couscous, sweet and white potatoes, white rice, and breakfast cereals like Cream of Wheat and Mini-Wheats.
- **High glycemic index (GI 70 or above):** Bagels, croissants, white and whole wheat breads, rice cakes, cakes, most crackers, doughnuts, and most packaged breakfast cereals.

The glycemic load is a little more difficult. Glycemic loads are figured by taking into account how much fiber and carbohydrates are in a food, and then determining how much the food will spike a person's blood sugar.

- **Low glycemic load (10 or less):** Most fruits and vegetables, meats without additives, whole grain breads, beans, and nuts have a low glycemic load
- **Moderate glycemic load (10-19):** Most packaged breakfast cereals, dried fruits, grapes, bananas, whole grain pastas, steel cut oats, and pretzels
- **High glycemic load (20 or more):** Potatoes, pizza, most pastas, corn, instant oatmeal, and bagels

Ideally, a food will have both a low GI rating and a low GL rating to be considered a good choice for weight loss. However, that's not always the case. A food like watermelon may have a high glycemic index, at 76, but the glycemic load is a very low 5. This makes the watermelon an acceptable choice. A doughnut with the same 76 glycemic index has a higher glycemic load at 17, and added fats, making it a very poor food choice. If in doubt about glycemic loads, a chart has been provided in the last chapter. This is also a number that is easily found with a quick internet search. If in doubt, it is always best to search for both the glycemic index and the glycemic load of a food.

Foods that have low glycemic values tend to be low fat and minimally processed, so choosing foods based on their glycemic index level may help with weight management.

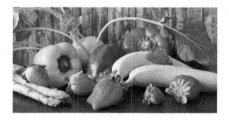

A low-glycemic diet may provide some people with the necessary guidance to help them make better choices for a healthy meal plan. However, the glycemic index and glycemic loads are not to be used in isolation—factors such as calories, fat, fiber, vitamins, and other nutrients should be taken into account.

But wait a minute—if you don't know which foods are causing you to gain weight in the first place, how can you lose weight? Some foods you eat on a daily basis appear to be harmless but are actually responsible for the rising number on your scale. On the surface, some of these foods appear to be healthy, which means you may be eating more of them than you would normally allow yourself for unhealthy foods. Eating too many calories, even if they are from healthy foods, will contribute to weight gain, as mentioned in Chapter 1.

Here is a quick list of these foods:

- **Breakfast cereals:** These are laden with sugar; some do have dietary fiber but only in small quantities. Even low sugar breakfast cereals are often manufactured using flours that quickly convert to sugar in the bloodstream.
- **Canned and cream-based soups:** These are high in sodium, which may result in bloating and water retention. Cream based soups are often loaded with fat, which will likely contribute to weight gain.
- **Fruit juice:** Turning fruit into juice strips it of fiber, and the sugar levels in the concentrated liquid are as high as those in soda. To get more fiber and vitamins, eat your fruit whole. Also, research suggests that some fruits, such as strawberries, raspberries, and blueberries, are high in polyphenols, which are natural chemicals that can prevent fat formation, rendering them more effective than others at fighting belly fat.
- **Bottled fruit smoothies:** A fruit smoothie may appear to be a healthy option, but many store-bought bottled smoothies are just bulked-up fruit juices with little fiber. Some contain

up to 440 calories, which is nearly a third of what the average woman on a 1,500-calorie weight-loss diet requires per day.

Additionally, many of our favorite foods have excitotoxins. These are nonessential amino acids that stimulate savory taste buds and fool our brain into thinking the food is more flavorful than it really is. This may lead to overeating even when we're full. So, it's not lack of self-control that makes you keep reaching for that pack of chicken-flavored crackers—it's excitotoxins. The following are regarded as some of the most harmful excitotoxins:

- Monosodium glutamate (MSG) is a flavor enhancer that is added to many foods such as processed foods, soups, fast foods, and canned foods.
- Aspartame is a widely used low-calorie artificial sweetener.
- Domoic acid is a naturally occurring nonessential amino acid.
- Cysteine is produced industrially by hydrolysis and is important in the production of meaty and savory artificial flavors.

Let's take a closer look at two of the most commonly known excitotoxins: MSG and aspartame.

According to research, one of the possible negative effects of MSG is weight gain. People who started a trial at a healthy weight but were taking in around 5 grams per day were 33% more likely to be overweight at the end of the research 5 years later (He et al., 2011). What's shocking is that this weight gain is independent of caloric consumption. Researchers are of the view that the MSG dietary additive may interfere with the signaling abilities of appetite-regulating hormones.

Artificial sweeteners such as aspartame were created as a sugar alternative to aid in the reduction of insulin resistance and obesity. However, research shows that their effects may contribute to an increase in body mass index (BMI) and the development of metabolic syndrome. Artificial sweeteners appear to modify the host micro-biota, diminish satiety, and disrupt glucose homeostasis, and they are linked to increased calorie consumption and weight gain.

Planning and preparing your meals ahead of time will make it possible for you to avoid foods with additives that may sabotage your health and weight-loss efforts.

Must-Haves in a Good Weight-Loss Meal Plan

Now let's take a look at what a good weight-loss meal plan should look like.

Protein

According to research, higher-protein diets are good for achieving fat reduction and improving body-weight control because protein does the following:

- controls your appetite by making you feel full longer with less food
- helps increase and maintain muscle mass
- lowers the risk of bone fractures and osteoporosis as you age
- increases your metabolism, helping you burn more calories
- helps lower your blood pressure and cholesterol and lowers the risk of stroke, heart attack, and kidney disease

The American College of Sports Medicine recommends 0.36 grams of protein per pound of body weight, or 0.8 grams of protein per kilogram of body weight, to maintain muscle. This is 54 grams of protein for a 150-pound individual. An ounce of cooked meat has around 7 grams of protein, so if a person weighs 150 pounds, they should eat roughly 8 ounces of meat throughout the day. If more protein is required, add healthy alternatives such as 1% cottage cheese or fat-free plain Greek yogurt with fruit for dessert. Some dishes can even be made vegan by substituting vegan ingredients.

In a study published by the Oxford Academic, researchers analyzed the data from several studies and found that measuring the amount of protein one eats at every meal to ensure adequate protein consumption not only positively impacted the overall health of participants, but was a significant factor in weight reduction. Eating the proper amount of protein is a critical foundation for weight control.

Fiber

Research also indicates that foods high in soluble fiber help reduce and remove belly fat. Foods with soluble fiber include beans, apples, peas, carrots, broccoli, avocados, and citrus fruit. When soluble fiber combines with water, it forms a gel-like substance that slows the rate at which the stomach releases digested food into the intestine; this prevents constipation, makes you feel fuller, and lowers blood sugar levels and cholesterol.

In an analysis of several weight loss studies, researchers found that an increase of fruits and vegetables in the diet increased weight loss. A more interesting finding was that the increase of fruits and vegetables contributed to the weight loss of women more so than the weight loss of the men. Fruits and vegetables are an important way to add fiber to your weight loss program.

Omega 3 Fatty Acids

The body doesn't manufacture omega-3 fatty acids, but it needs them to maintain optimum health. Omega-3 fatty acids are a type of polyunsaturated healthy fat found in fish oil that may aid in weight loss because they help curb appetite and hunger. In one study, two groups of healthy people on a weight-loss diet were asked to consume fish oil omega-3 each day. One group consumed 0.3 grams and the other 1.3 grams. The group that consumed 1.3 grams reported feeling significantly fuller for up to 2 hours after a meal (Parra et al., 2008).

These effects, however, are not universal.

In another small study, two groups of healthy adults not on a weight-loss diet were given 5 grams of fish oil and a placebo every day, respectively. The group given fish oil reported having a 28% stronger desire to eat and feeling about 20% less full after eating a regular breakfast (Damsbo-Svendsen et al., 2013).

What's interesting here is that one study found that fish oil omega-3 increased levels of a fullness hormone in obese people while the other study found these levels decreased in non-obese people given fish oil omega-3.

So, the possibility exists that the effects of fish oil omega-3 may vary depending on your health and diet. More research is needed, however, before firm conclusions can be drawn. Omega-3 is found in foods such as seeds, brussels sprouts, tuna, and nuts.

Vitamin C

Most of us know vitamin C as an immunity booster, but it is also an antioxidant, making it even more important when people who are overweight or obese are attempting to lose weight. Any weight gain can cause inflammation, thus increasing the production of free radicals, causing a chain reaction of hormonal and metabolic effects such as insulin resistance that may encourage further weight gain. So, consuming sufficient antioxidants is important in the prevention of inflammation-related weight gain, and research indicates that overweight people have higher needs due to higher free radical production. Foods that are high in vitamin C include broccoli, kale, Brussels sprouts, kiwi, lemon, orange, and chili pepper.

Magnesium

Many different enzyme systems, including those involved in metabolism and glucose regulation, require magnesium for reactions to occur, and research suggests a direct link between insulin resistance and magnesium intake. Insulin resistance, as mentioned earlier, can make it difficult for many people to lose weight. Consuming enough magnesium every day can gradually reduce insulin resistance and may be a key component of a weight-loss plan. Foods that are rich in magnesium include spinach, broccoli, edamame, bananas, leafy greens, tuna, and yogurt.

There's no one-size-fits-all fat-reduction plan, so when planning your meals, you should keep your specific needs in mind, like the following, for instance:

- how much weight you need to shed in order to increase your exercise levels
- any dietary needs due to medical conditions
- any dietary needs that are personal, cultural, or religious
- how much time you have for shopping and meal preparation
- your cooking abilities as well as the difficulty or simplicity of the recipes
- whether additional members of the household should be included in the meal plan

3

CHOOSING THE PLAN THAT'S RIGHT FOR YOU

Contrary to popular belief, there are numerous ways to meal prep without spending an entire afternoon over the weekend cooking dishes for the upcoming week. To succeed in your weight-loss efforts, you need to choose a meal-prep plan that is right for you and your needs and that can be easily slotted into your schedule. Have another look at the list of things to consider when creating a meal plan in the previous chapter.

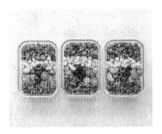

The most difficult part of meal planning for most of us is factoring in our social life. In my experience, most people take an all-or-nothing approach to meal prep, which makes it unsustainable in the long run. Make a note of when you're likely to eat out, and plan your meal-prep time with this in mind. For example, if you know you'll be out to dinner with friends on weekends, don't prepare meals for those nights. Your lifestyle should determine your approach.

In this book we are going to talk about four tried and tested meal plans:

Once-and-done

- **Once-and-done meal-prep plan:** If you do not have time to cook a meal each evening, this plan gives you the convenience of simply heating up what has been cooked in advance. The benefit of this plan is that portions can be weighed ahead of time, making it easier to stick to a weight-loss plan. An essential component of this plan is creating distinctly different meals for the week, ensuring that you are not eating the same thing day after day. If you do not like leftovers or food that has been cooked and then frozen, this will not work for you. Also, this plan requires a lot of freezer space.

Power Hour

- **Power-hour meal-prep plan:** If you prefer cooking daily and are willing to spend about a half hour in the evenings prepping your meals, this plan could work for you. This plan requires spending a little over an hour preparing ahead the main ingredients for your meals, so you will spend less time in the kitchen and get your meals to the table sooner. This is a good plan if you do not have hours to spend on meal prepping over the weekend.

Batch Prepping

- **Batch-prepping plan:** This involves preparing large

amounts of food at one time and freezing them raw in labeled containers. This allows you to simply pull from the prepared batches to swiftly create meals throughout the week. The key to making this plan work is organization, containers, labeling, and sufficient freezer space. This plan will save you time and money if you are diligent about keeping to your portion sizes.

Hybrid

- **Hybrid meal-prep plan:** This involves taking some elements from each of the above three plans to create a new plan. Some meals will be cooked during your prep, some meals will be prepared to be cooked later in the week, and some meals will be batch-prepped to use at a later date.

We will discuss these meal-prep plans thoroughly in the coming chapters.

The idea of meal prepping is to help you use efficiently the little time you have in the kitchen. Before you get into any of the three meal-prep plans, the following needs to be in place:

- Make a detailed list of your meals for the coming week or month. You could even make a weekly menu plan, such as fish on Monday, chili on Tuesday, casserole on Wednesday, and so forth. It can make planning easier, and it works particularly well if you have children because they like knowing what to expect. This list will help you when compiling your grocery list. Also, be sure to check your kitchen and be sure you have all the spices, herbs and condiments you will need for all your meals. There are weekly planning sheets for each plan at the end of each plan's chapter.
- Choose a day each week to prepare as many of your dishes as

possible. If you are batch prepping, choose a day on the weekend. Play some music and make it enjoyable. Invite a friend over to help with the work and the cooking, creating meals for two families in one day. Make it a family affair by assigning everyone a job that is appropriate for their age.

- To make the task more enjoyable and stress-free, make sure you have the right tools for the job.

Before we get into the individual meal-prep plans, let's discuss the basic tools and equipment needed to help make meal prep a breeze.

Basic Equipment

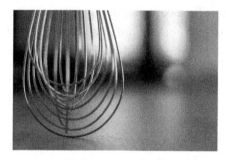

Like any other activity, you need to have the right tools to do a proper job. Meal prepping is no different. These are the basic tools you need for a seamless, dare I say pleasant, meal-prepping experience.

In addition to the basics of spoons, spatulas, storage bags, labels, and dishcloths, the following are some important items to have on hand.

- **Knife set**

Sharp knives are probably the most important tools you need to have for food prep. When you have the right knives, chopping becomes considerably easier and more effective.

But I would say the most important knife to have is a really good, steady chef's knife. Choose one that fits comfortably in your hand

and isn't too heavy.

- **Cutting boards**

Having multiple cutting boards on hand is highly recommended—one for vegetables, one for raw meat, and one for raw chicken. Choose a large cutting board that can accommodate all the vegetables you'll be chopping; wooden cutting boards are great for vegetables. For the meats, I suggest plastic cutting boards because they are not as porous as wooden ones and blood will not seep into the board.

- **Measuring cups and spoons**

These are great when following recipes, especially those that require measuring liquids.

- **Scale**

Some recipes require weight measurements, so having this on hand is useful—especially if you're a baker. Food scales are also useful for understanding portion amounts and measuring your food intake.

- **Air fryer**

An air fryer can cook almost anything that would normally be fried in oil, such as onion rings, chicken nuggets, and chicken fingers. Another great thing about an air fryer is that it doesn't heat up the kitchen the way an oven can.

- **Slow cooker**

Making meal preparation as quick and easy as possible requires efficiency. Electric slow cookers, sometimes known as crock pots, are very useful. You can cook anything from soup to pork loin in a slow cooker during the day and have it ready for your evening meal.

- **Pots and Pans**

The best way to cook food in bulk is using sheet pans and making one-pot meals. You'll be able to prepare enough food for lunches and dinners, and because it all comes together in one pan or pot, there isn't much cleaning up to do.

Non-rimmed sheet pans are fantastic for baking cookies while rimmed sheet pans are great for roasting vegetables and creating sheet pan dinners. If any liquid is leaked during cooking, the rim prevents it from dripping all over your oven and making a major mess.

- **Meat thermometer**

A meat thermometer is a helpful tool for ensuring that meat is cooked perfectly every time. Get one that allows you to monitor your meat from a distance or, better still, one that allows you to monitor the meat from your phone for a true hands-off experience.

- **A gadget that chops and blends**

Many different types of these are on the market—get one that's great for chopping, blending, and shredding. You can use it for making sauces, cauliflower rice, salsas, and so forth.

- **Mixing bowls**

Having a couple bowls available is useful for meal preparation and cooking in general. Even better if they have lids, because they'll do double duty and be useful as storage containers as well.

- **Casserole dishes**

These are obviously for making casseroles, and it helps to have them in various sizes. These dishes are also great for roasts and anything else you may bake.

- **Food-storage containers**

You may store your prepared food in any container you have on hand, but I prefer glass, as it does not leach hazardous chemicals into your food the way certain plastics do, and reheating in the microwave and on the stove is easy. If you have a storage set, everything will match, and it will be easier to store—otherwise, you'll wind up with a wild cabinet full of mismatched storage containers that come falling out every time you open the cabinet.

Use clear storage containers so you can see what's inside. This is especially useful when you have small children—they can see the already-cut-up fruit without opening every container.

- **Mason jars**

These are great not just for meal prepping but also for packing work lunches and salads.

- **Dish towels**

You will need these to clean up as you go and when you are done prepping. These can also be placed under plastic chopping boards to keep them from shifting while you're chopping.

- **Aluminum foil and/or parchment paper**

These are great for lining pans so you can quickly and easily wash them after every use. Aluminum foil is also great for creating packets to keep your food warm.

Suitable Foods for Meal Prepping

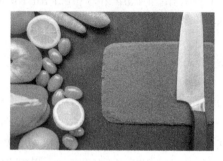

Not all foods are suitable for meal prepping; some foods need to be eaten soon after preparation, and others lose their nutritional efficacy if frozen. The following foods are suitable for meal prepping:

- **Frozen vegetables:** Brussels sprouts, peas, cauliflower, green beans, broccoli, riced vegetables, cauliflower pizza crust
- **Starchy vegetables:** parsnip, yuca, cassava
- **Stiff fresh vegetables:** celery, radishes, carrots, cabbage, bell peppers
- **Sturdy greens:** kale, spinach
- **Legumes:** chickpeas, beans, lentils, peas
- **Lean protein:** eggs, frozen or canned seafood, shredded cheese, lean cuts of meat
- **Whole fruit:** apples, bananas, oranges, clementines, plums, peaches, pears
- **Nuts and seeds:** almonds, peanuts, walnuts, pumpkin seeds, flax, chia

Depending on the ingredients, prepared foods can be refrigerated for 2–5 days or frozen for 3–4 months. Keep cold food at temperatures below 40 °F and hot foods above 140 °F to be safe and avoid food-borne illnesses. Sealing food in airtight packaging or storage containers not only keeps bacteria out but also preserves flavor and locks in moisture.

Sometimes with meal prepping, storage can become a challenge. Fortunately, there are some fruits and vegetables that do not require refrigeration:

- tomatoes
- sweet potatoes
- garlic
- onions
- avocados
- pears
- apples
- bananas
- limes and lemons
- oranges

Pantry Staples

Keeping a stock of pantry staples on hand is an excellent way to streamline your meal-prep process and make menu creation easier.

Here are a few versatile and healthy foods to keep in your pantry:

- **Canned goods:** low-sodium broth, tomatoes, tomato sauce, tuna, chicken, spaghetti sauce, salsa, green chilis, tomato and green chili blend
- **Oils:** cooking spray
- **Spices:** salt, pepper, chili powder, smoked paprika, garlic powder, onion powder, Italian seasoning
- **Other:** pea protein powder, rice protein powder, sugar substitute

4

ONCE-AND-DONE MEAL-PREP PLAN

The once-and-done meal-prep plan is good for people who don't have time to prepare and cook their meals during the week. This plan allows you to prepare a variety of precooked meals for the entire week in 3–4 hours.

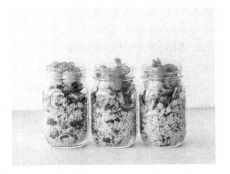

Food that will be eaten within 5 days should be stored in the refrigerator, and the rest of the food should be stored in the freezer and thawed a day or two before it will be eaten.

For meal-prepping to work, planning is key. Important to note is that planning is not just about the meals; it includes the equipment and tools needed for making meal preparation a breeze. Before we get into the activity part, you need to have all your tools and equipment lined up and within easy reach. Trying to find things once you have started with your prep is not fun.

So, for the once-and-done meal-prep plan, start by sourcing a few recipes that are hands off and an equal number of recipes that are hands on. Hands-off recipes are those that require baking or roasting in the oven, steaming, and air frying. These are recipes that require minimal monitoring—you just turn the heat and the timer on and leave them alone. Hands-on recipes, on the other hand, need monitoring, such as stirring and turning over; these are typically cooked on the stove—boiling and sautéing, for example.

Decide on possible methods to prepare the proteins, such as Instant Pot, slow cooker, oven, air fryer, and stove top. Everything will be made in one day. If making a slow cooker meal, that will be cooked on high for an hour and then switch to low for the remainder of the day so that it is ready when dinnertime arrives. Ensure there's enough liquid in the slow cooker, and use a liner for easy cleanup.

Not everyone likes spending time in the kitchen, and most people dread cleaning up. To reduce time spent on cleaning up, use aluminum foil or parchment to line cookie sheets, oven pans, muffin tins, and cake pans. You can also place sautéed vegetables and roasted meats in aluminum foil packets on the countertop to cool while you move onto the next dish. This way you can reuse the same pan over and over. Fill the sink with soapy water and toss dishes and utensils in the water as you use them. You can easily rinse and re-use the same items this way, and when you are done, they will be ready to rinse or toss into the dishwasher.

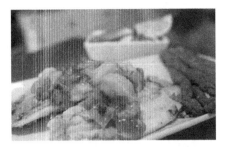

Mango Salsa Tilapia

A varied diet increases the diversity of beneficial bacteria in your digestive tract, helping you maintain a healthy weight and also improving the efficiency of your immune system. Most importantly, rotating your ingredients will ensure you don't eat the same thing over and over, because that could result in you reaching for something that could undo some of your good work. Rotating your ingredients is critical for weight reduction.

For a weight-reduction plan that calls for breakfast, you will need to make sure you have six different primary proteins and fruits. Only four primary proteins and fruits are required if a diet involves intermittent fasting.

Opt for dishes that will make it easy for you to rotate four to six additional lean, unprocessed, clean protein ingredients such as pork loin, halibut, 93% beef, edamame, 1% cottage cheese, filet mignon, egg whites, sirloin, chicken breast, plain unsweetened low-fat yogurt, protein powder, turkey breast, tempeh, tofu, cod, tuna, and tilapia.

For lunches and dinners, choose no more than three low-glycemic-index vegetables such as peppers and onions to prepare. The rest of the vegetables, such as fresh green beans, or spaghetti squash, can be cooked whole—or you can use frozen vegetables, which can be cooked in the microwave while you are busy with the rest of the preparations.

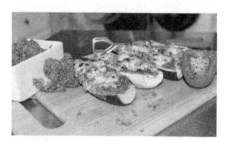

Lasagna Boats

Include no more than two low-glycemic-index fruits, like melons, oranges, and cranberries to be prepped by cooking, cutting, segmenting, peeling, or destemming, for example. The rest of the fruit can be eaten whole, like plums, apples, pears, and so forth.

Find recipes for each protein; it will save time if all the oven or air fryer recipes require the same temperature. Choose three stove-top protein recipes per week, such as sweet chili pork or breakfast sausage. Stove-top dishes take time because they need to be stirred and attended to, but many items may be prepared while a dish is cooking in the oven. Preparing more than one casserole-style meal each week will require significantly more effort in the kitchen, so try to limit your menu to one.

Create a planner and grocery list, taking your dietary needs into consideration. Frozen vegetables and fresh meat both cook out around one third of their weight. So, if 6 ounces of chicken is required per serving, cook approximately 9 ounces of raw chicken for each dish. Raw vegetables lose nearly a quarter of their weight when cooked, so if 6 ounces of cooked squash is required per serving, start with around 8 ounces of raw squash.

Now let's plan the prep step by step:

1. Preheat the oven. Ensure that the dishwasher and trash can are empty and the sink is filled with warm soapy water. This

will aid in cleaning up throughout the preparation process, saving time.

2. Before preparing any food, place all the vegetables that need to be baked, such as spaghetti squash, tomatillos, and so forth, on a cookie sheet lined with foil, and place them in the oven.

3. Prepare the marinades and spice mixes that you'll be using, and set aside to allow the flavors to blend.

4. Next, prepare all the fresh fruits and vegetables, and set aside on paper plates or aluminum foil.

5. Prepare all the meats that are to be marinated, and put them in the marinades.

6. Meals such as pork loin and meat loaf take a long time to cook, so they should be prepared next and put in the oven, slow cooker, or air fryer to cook.

7. Meals like lasagna boats and stuffed bell peppers that cook like a casserole should follow. Prepare them and get them into the oven.

8. The next meal to be prepared is the meal that needs to be simmered on the stovetop—chili or spaghetti, for example. This should be placed on the stovetop to simmer while the other meals cook.

9. Get the oven-baked breakfast ready, and place it in the oven to cook.

10. Next up is the first stove-top dinner/lunch meal. Once cooked, set it aside on foil or in a separate bowl to cool down as you will need the pan.

11. Put together the ingredients for the stove-top breakfast, and cook in a separate pan while keeping an eye on the first stove-top dinner/lunch.

12. Once the first stove-top dinner/lunch and the stove-top breakfast are cooked, clean the pan, and start cooking the second stove-top dinner/lunch meal.

13. While you cook the stove-top meals, keep an eye on the food

that's cooking in the oven and remove these foods to cool as they finish cooking.

14. Remember to clean up as you go.
15. Once everything is cooked, portion out the food into labeled containers for the week.

Before putting the food in the refrigerator or freezer, allow it to cool down completely. Food should not sit out for longer than 2 hours.

Here's the once-and-done meal-prep plan process summary:

- You need to choose four to six proteins for the week. This is dependent on your weight-loss program. Make sure that half the meals are oven baked, meaning hands off; the other half should be stove top. All the meals should be cooked on the day of the prep and warmed up as needed throughout the week.
- Next, choose the vegetables that will go with each protein. Prepare no more than three fresh vegetables. The rest of the vegetables should be jarred, canned, or frozen.
- Choose fruits that will be eaten cooked and those that will be eaten fresh with each meal. Aim to prep no more than two types of fruit, such as cooked blueberries to be poured over pancakes, and peeled and segmented mandarin oranges or cut cantaloupe, for example.

Sample Once-and-Done Prep Day

SAMPLE ONCE-AND-DONE MEAL PREP PLANNER		
PROTEINS	**VEGETABLES**	**FRUITS**
PROTEIN 1: Beef **RECIPE:** Beef with broccoli stir-fry	frozen broccoli onion (prep)	peach (fresh)
PROTEIN 2: Fish **RECIPE:** Mango-salsa tilapia	bell peppers (prep) onion (prep) jalapeño (prep)	mango (prep)
PROTEIN 3: Pork **RECIPE:** Pork loin roast	frozen asparagus jarred mushrooms	applesauce (jarred)
PROTEIN 4: Turkey **RECIPE:** Turkey chili	canned tomatoes bell pepper (prep) onion (prep)	orange (fresh)
PROTEIN 5: Pea protein powder **RECIPE:** Protein pancakes	n/a	Blueberries (frozen)
PROTEIN 6: Rice protein powder **RECIPE:** Pumpkin spice cookies	canned pumpkin	Strawberries (prep)

1. Choose six proteins for variety.
2. Choose recipes to go with the proteins you have chosen.
3. Choose vegetables to go with each recipe (no more than 3 to prep, the rest canned, jarred, or frozen).
4. Choose the fruits to eat with each meal (no more than 2 to prep, the rest canned, jarred, or frozen).
5. Create a grocery list.

GROCERIES

1 lb. sirloin	
1 lb. fish	
1 lb. pork loin roast	
1 lb. ground turkey	
Pea protein powder	
Rice protein powder	
3 onions	
1 jalapeño	
3 red bell peppers	
melon	
1 mango	
peach	
blueberries	
strawberries	
frozen asparagus	
frozen broccoli	
stewed tomatoes	
canned pumpkin	
jarred mushrooms	
egg whites	
sweetener	
spices	

For a printable version of all the sample and blank planners, scan the QR code or email us at brooksmealprepbooks@gmail.com

The purpose of the sample prep day is to show you how to work the plan with six proteins. If you are doing intermittent fasting, work with four proteins. For this example, we will use breakfast cookies, protein pancakes, broccoli beef stir fry, pork loin, turkey chili, and mango salsa tilapia.

Although this plan is the most complicated, when you follow these guidelines, it should take less than 4 hours from start to finish:

Planning the Day

Choose six proteins for variety. This sample day needs the following proteins:

- ground turkey
- pork loin
- fish
- sirloin
- rice protein powder
- pea protein powder

Choose recipes to go with the proteins you have chosen. All of your meals for the week will be cooked during your once-and-done prep. This sample day includes the following recipes:

- Broccoli and Beef Stir Fry
- Pork Loin Roast
- Mango-Salsa Tilapia
- Turkey Chili
- Protein Pancakes
- Pumpkin Spice Cookies

Choose vegetables to go with each recipe. You should choose no more than three fresh vegetables to prep, the rest should be canned, jarred, or frozen. This sample day includes the following prepped vegetables:

- three onions
- three bell peppers
- one jalapeño

Choose the fruits to eat with each meal. You should choose no more than two fresh fruits to prep, the rest of the fruit should be canned, jarred, or frozen. This sample prep day includes the following prepped fruits:

- mango diced for salsa
- strawberries, destemmed and portioned

Create a grocery list. Look at all the ingredients for all the recipes to create this list. It's a terrible feeling to be in the middle of a great prep day and suddenly have everything come crashing to a halt because you are out of one ingredient. Take the time to be sure you have everything you need.

How the Once-and-Done Prep Will Look

1. Prepare the kitchen by filling the sink with soapy water, and emptying both the trashcan and dishwasher. Also, check to be sure you have all the utensils, gadgets and ingredients at hand.

2. Preheat your oven to 350°F and adjust the cook times to accommodate one temperature. You will cook for less time the recipes that call for a lower temperature and longer for recipes that require a higher temperature. Using one oven temperature for everything will save a lot of time.

3. If any of the vegetables need to be cooked whole in the oven, put them in the oven for roasting at this point. For this sample prep plan, we are not roasting whole vegetables.

4. Create the spice mixes and marinades and set aside. You will need spices for searing the pork loin and a marinade for the broccoli beef

stir fry. For the tilapia, you'll need only salt and pepper, and the spices for the chili will be added while cooking.

5. Prepare all vegetables and all fruits before starting on the meat.

- Slice and dice the onions.
- Slice the red bell peppers.
- Chop up the jalapeño.
- Dice the mango, and combine it with all ingredients but the cilantro. Place the cilantro in cold water to bring out its flavor.

6. Prepare the meats that need marinating, and place them in the marinade while you prepare the other meals. Fish will usually be plenty flavorful with just 15 minutes of marinating. For this sample plan, we will not marinate the fish, however, when marinating fish, do not marinate or longer than 30 minutes.

- Chop up the beef for the stir fry, and add it to the marinade with the diced onions.

7. Move on to the dish that will take the longest to cook; in this case, it's the pork loin.

- Prepare the pork loin according to the recipe, and place it in the oven. The safest way to ensure you don't overcook your pork loin is to use a meat thermometer that beeps when the pork loin is cooked through.

9. Next, prepare the stove-top dish; in this case, it is the turkey chili. Brown the meat with the spices. Place all remaining ingredients in the pot, and simmer for at least 20 minutes.

10. Now, move on to the oven-baked breakfast. For this sample day, we are using pumpkin-spiced breakfast cookies. Prepare the cookie

batter, and start baking the cookies in the oven along with the pork loin.

11. Next, move on to the beef for the stir fry. Cook the beef with the onions that you marinated earlier. In the meantime, mix the protein-pancake breakfast batter. When the beef has finished cooking, place it in foil or a bowl to cool down so you can use the same pan for the next marinated meat.

12. In a separate pan, cook the stove-top breakfast (protein pancakes). While washing the pan that you cooked the beef in, watch the pancakes so they don't burn.

13. Once the first stove-top breakfast is done cooking, cook the second stove-top dish, the tilapia, in the clean frying pan. While the fish is cooking, assemble the ingredients for the mango salsa.

When everything is cooked and has cooled down, place the foods into containers for reheating through the week.

At first the once-and-done meal-prep plan may seem complicated, but once you start, you'll find your rhythm, and everything will flow.

I've included a blank planning chart to help you get started.

ONCE-AND-DONE MEAL PREP PLANNER			GROCERIES
PROTEINS	**VEGETABLES**	**FRUITS**	
PROTEIN 1: **RECIPE:**			
PROTEIN 2: **RECIPE:**			
PROTEIN 3: **RECIPE:**			
PROTEIN 4: **RECIPE:**			
PROTEIN 5: **RECIPE:**			
PROTEIN 6: **RECIPE:**			

1. Choose six proteins for variety.
2. Choose recipes to go with the proteins you have chosen.
3. Choose vegetables to go with each recipe (no more than 3 to prep, the rest canned, jarred, or frozen).
4. Choose the fruits to eat with each meal (no more than 2 to prep, the rest canned, jarred, or frozen).
5. Create a grocery list.

For a printable version of all the sample and blank planners, scan the QR code or email us at brooksmealprepbooks@gmail.com

5

THE POWER-HOUR MEAL-PREP PLAN

The power-hour meal-prep plan is a great plan for when you don't have enough hours in a day but can afford to spare at least an hour for meal prepping. I say "at least" because realistically you'll need an hour and a half, especially if breakfasts are part of your meal prep. Be prepared to use your stove, and oven or air fryer. Although the power hour will go by quickly, many of your cooking gadgets and equipment have a place in this plan. Remember to gather all the equipment and tools needed for meal prepping, as listed in Chapter 3.

When I prep using this plan, I prepare four dinners to cook when I get home, and plan to go out to eat one night during the week. I also make enough for dinner to ensure I have leftovers to take for my lunches throughout the week. In this way, the plan provides all of my meals for the days I work.

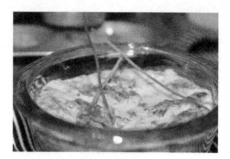

Omelet Muffins

The planning for the power-hour meal prep goes like this:

1. Prepare all the dinner proteins and vegetables for the week in advance so that they are ready to cook whenever they are required. Prepare two breakfasts to eat on alternate days during the week. You could also prepare lunches instead of breakfasts. Or, if you don't like the idea of taking leftovers for lunch, once you get the hang of it you could prepare both lunches and breakfasts during your power hour prep.

2. Choose two dishes to cook that will taste great reheated during your power hour - chili, muffins, or meatballs for example.

3. Choose only one of the following: one constructed protein dish, such as a casserole, or one stovetop simmering dish, such as chili, or meat spaghetti sauce.

4. Choose one or two protein-and-vegetable dishes, such as fajitas

5. Choose one or two meals with meat prepared whole to be baked or grilled, such as barbecue chicken

6. Choose one breakfast to be baked during prepping and another to be prepped and cooked on the morning it will be needed or cooked the night before.

Remember, rotating your ingredients is helpful for weight reduction, and research has supported the idea of doing this at least every two days. I also find it nicer to have variety throughout the week. So, six different primary proteins and fruits will be required. If your diet involves intermittent fasting, only four primary proteins and fruits will be required for food rotation.

Now let's plan for the prep:

Select recipes that will allow you to rotate four to six lean, unprocessed, excitotoxin-free proteins. You can choose lean proteins such as pork loin, 93% beef, 1% cottage cheese, edamame, egg whites, filet mignon, sirloin, protein powder, chicken breast, turkey breast, tofu, tempeh, cod, halibut, tilapia, tuna, plain unsweetened low-fat Greek yogurt, and so forth.

Complete a planner sheet and grocery list based on the recipes you have chosen.

The following activities will take place on the prep day:

1. Place all marinade and spice ingredients in labeled, plastic freezer storage bags and set aside. You will get the food ready while the spices meld together.

2. Prepare all of the vegetables. Vegetables that need to be cooked at the same time as meats should be chopped and added to those meats —for fajitas, for example. Prepare other vegetables, such as zucchini spirals, and store them.

3. Peel, cut, destem, and weigh all the fruits that will be required for the week. Store them in glass containers, and they will stay fresh longer.

4. Mix together all the ingredients required for an oven-baked breakfast, such as omelet muffins, quiche, cheesecake, and so forth, and place them in oven-friendly glass containers. This will make it easy for you to quickly toss them in the oven while getting ready in the morning or during dinner the night before.

5. Next, mix the ingredients for breakfasts that need to be cooked on the stove top, like omelets and pancakes. When you are done mixing, portion the mixture into plastic bags that are small enough to allow you to easily pour the mixture into a pan for cooking in the morning. If you have extra time, you can also quickly cook this dish during your power hour prep and freeze what will not be eaten within the next few days.

6. Chop and weigh out all the proteins and tenderize those that will benefit from the process. Place all the proteins into the plastic freezer storage bags with the marinades, add fresh vegetables (if using) into the bags, and seal the bags. This method works well with pork and beef as well as onions and bell peppers, but proteins like fish and poultry may take on too much of the marinade flavor and shouldn't be marinated as long. Fish should marinate no longer than 30 minutes and poultry for anywhere from four to 24 hours. Prepare the fish or poultry marinade during the power hour and place it in a zip storage bag so it's ready when it's time to marinate. Most vegetables will break down when marinated, so stick to onions and peppers.

7. Depending on when the meals will be eaten, place the sealed bags into the freezer or refrigerator.

8. This is a good time to form things like meatballs, if making.

9. While you prepare the week of food, you may also select a recipe that is the quickest to cook, and cook a meal for the following day's lunch.

Here's the power hour meal-prep plan process summary:

- You need to choose four to six proteins for the week. This is dependent on your weight-loss program. Two of the meals should be cooked on the day of the prep and should utilize recipes that taste great warmed up when needed throughout the week.

- Next, choose the vegetables that will go with each protein. Prepare no more than three fresh vegetables. The rest of the vegetables should be jarred, canned, or frozen.
- Choose fruits that will be eaten with each meal. Aim to prep no more than two types of fruit, such as cooked blueberries to be poured over pancakes, and peeled and segmented mandarin oranges or cut cantaloupe, for example.

Sample Power Hour Prep Day

SAMPLE POWER HOUR MEAL PREP PLANNER			GROCERIES	
PROTEINS	VEGETABLES	FRUITS		
PROTEIN 1: Turkey RECIPE: Turkey Chili	Canned tomatoes bell pepper (prep) onion (prep)	melon (prep)	1 lb. turkey	
			1 lb. pork loin	
PROTEIN 2: Pork RECIPE: Pork Loin Roast	jarred sauerkraut	strawberries (prep)	1 lb. chicken breasts	
			1 lb. sirloin	
			rice protein powder	
			1% cottage cheese	
PROTEIN 3: Chicken RECIPE: BBQ Chicken	frozen green beans	pear (fresh)	3 bell peppers	
			2 onions	
			melon	
PROTEIN 4: Beef RECIPE: Beef Fajitas	peppers (prep) onions (prep)	peaches (canned)	strawberries	
			pears	
			applesauce	
			peaches	
PROTEIN 5: Rice Protein Powder RECIPE: Chocolate Muffins	n/a	applesauce (jarred)	frozen cherries	
			frozen green beans	
			canned tomatoes	
PROTEIN 6: Cottage Cheese RECIPE: Breakfast Cheesecakes	n/a	cherries (frozen)	jarred mushrooms	
			jarred sauerkraut	
			egg whites	
1. Choose six proteins for variety.			cocoa powder	
2. Choose recipes to go with the proteins you have chosen (2 that will taste great reheated & cook in 1 hr.).			sweetener	
3. Choose vegetables to go with each recipe (no more than 3 to prep, the rest canned, jarred, or frozen).			sugar free ketchup	
4. Choose the fruits to eat with each meal (no more than 2 to prep, the rest canned, jarred, or frozen).			apple cider vinegar	
5. Create a grocery list.			spices	

For a printable version of all the sample and blank planners, scan the QR code or email us at brooksmealprepbooks@gmail.com

The purpose of the sample prep day is to show you how to work the plan with six proteins. If you are doing intermittent fasting, you can work with four proteins. For this example, we will use breakfast cheesecakes, chocolate muffins, turkey chili, pork loin, barbecue chicken, and beef fajitas.

This is the fastest plan for getting all your meals prepped and ready to cook throughout the week. This plan is commonly referred to as the power hour plan, but it will typically take a little more than an hour to complete. You will complete a planner using the steps that follow.

Planning the Day

1. Choose six proteins for variety. This sample day needs the following proteins:

- ground turkey
- pork loin
- chicken breasts
- sirloin
- rice protein powder
- cottage cheese

2. Choose recipes to go with the proteins you have chosen. Two proteins should be used for recipes that will taste great reheated & can be cooked in one hour. You will cook these two proteins during your power hour prep. This sample day includes the following recipes:

- Turkey Chili (cooked during prepping)
- Pork Loin Roast
- Barbecue Chicken
- Beef Fajitas
- Chocolate Muffins (cooked during prepping)
- Breakfast Cheesecakes

3. Choose vegetables to go with each recipe. You should choose no more than three fresh vegetables to prep, the rest should be canned, jarred, or frozen. This sample day includes the following prepped vegetables:

- onions
- bell peppers

4. Choose the fruits to eat with each meal. You should choose no more than two fresh fruits to prep, the rest of the fruit should be canned, jarred, or frozen. This sample prep day includes the following prepped fruits:

- melon, diced and portioned
- strawberries, destemmed and portioned

5. Create a grocery list. Look at all the ingredients for all the recipes to create this list. It's a terrible feeling to be in the middle of a great prep day and suddenly have everything come crashing to a halt because you've run out of one ingredient. Take the time to be sure you have everything you need.

How the Power Hour Prep Will Look

1. Start by preheating the oven if needed and while the oven is heating, fill the sink with soapy water and ensure the trashcan and dishwasher are empty so you can clean as you go

2. Prep the first item you will cook today and get it into the oven or onto the stove – the turkey chili for this sample day. If vegetables will be added to the dish – like onions and peppers, it is okay to start the dish cooking and add the vegetables later. Just get this dish started.

3. Next, prepare the second item you will cook today and get it into the oven or onto the stove – the chocolate muffins for this sample day.

4. Prepare all fresh fruits and vegetables at one time. This sample day needs the following vegetables prepped:

- three bell peppers for the fajitas and turkey chili
- two onions for the fajitas and turkey chili
- If your menu requires cooking some fruit, like frozen berries to pour over pancakes, start that item simmering on the stovetop before prepping any other fruits or vegetables. This sample day includes frozen cherries that can be cooked with sweetener and pre-portioned for the days to come.
- If the dishes you have started cooking today require fresh vegetables – like onions for the chili – prepare those vegetable first so they can start cooking with the meat. For this sample day, you will start on onions, and put into pot with meat. After you finish prepping all the onions, you will move on to the peppers, and add those as you finish dicing. Once those vegetables are sautéed to your preference, add the remaining chili ingredients.
- If needed, weigh out fruit portions for the week and place in zip storage bags or other containers. For this sample day, this step includes cubing and pre-portioning the melon, and de-stemming and pre-portioning the strawberries.
- Set aside all vegetables that will be combined with meats. For this sample prep day, the onions and bell peppers can be placed in the same gallon storage bag with the marinade and fajita meat.

5. Now, prepare all the marinades and dry spices you need for the week, and set aside in gallon storage bags. Let the flavors blend together while you prepare the remaining items for the day. For this sample day, you will prepare the dry rub for the pork loin, the barbecue sauce for the chicken, and the fajita marinade for the beef.

6. Prepare all meats by chopping, tenderizing, slicing, or dividing into portions. Add the meats to the marinades and spices, or place into

separate storage bag and store with marinade - depending on the recipe. For this sample day, place the chicken, beef, and pork loin into the same bags with the marinades and spices. All of these recipes do very well when frozen, and the meat is marinated while thawing.

7. Move on to the breakfast that will be baked in the morning while you get ready or baked the night before. Prepare the mixture and divide evenly into ramekins. For this sample day, you will prepare and pre-portion the breakfast cheesecakes.

8. As the chili and muffins are cooling, clean the kitchen.

At first, this plan may take you as long as two hours, but after only a couple of times, you will find that you are able to prepare all your meals for the week and have the entire kitchen clean in right around one hour. You can always shorten the time by only preparing the meals and cooking nothing during your prep.

I've included a blank planning chart to help you get started.

POWER HOUR MEAL PREP PLANNER			GROCERIES	
PROTEINS	VEGETABLES	FRUITS		
PROTEIN 1: RECIPE:				
PROTEIN 2: RECIPE:				
PROTEIN 3: RECIPE:				
PROTEIN 4: RECIPE:				
PROTEIN 5: RECIPE:				
PROTEIN 6: RECIPE:				

1. Choose six proteins for variety.
2. Choose recipes to go with the proteins you have chosen (2 that will taste great reheated & cook in 1 hr.).
3. Choose vegetables to go with each recipe (no more than 3 to prep, the rest canned, jarred, or frozen).
4. Choose the fruits to eat with each meal (no more than 2 to prep, the rest canned, jarred, or frozen).
5. Create a grocery list.

For a printable version of all the sample and blank planners, scan the QR code or email us at brooksmealprepbooks@gmail.com

6

THE BATCH-PREPPING PLAN

The batch-prepping meal-prep plan requires you to put aside 4-6 hours for prepping because you will be preparing meals for an entire month. It is best to do this over the weekend when you are not busy with other things.

The idea here is to use the same ingredients in multiple ways in different recipes throughout the month. What makes this great is that you prepare your ingredients only once a month, which allows you to buy in bulk and save money. The disadvantage of the batch-cooking meal plan is that it requires a lot of freezer space.

Before you get into it, remember to put out all the equipment and tools needed for meal prepping, as listed in Chapter 3. You don't want to be searching for equipment once you are in the swing of things.

- Choose four proteins, excluding breakfast items—many breakfast items are best left for weekly prep and will not be covered in this chapter. Once you are skilled at batch prepping, you can try your hand at recipes like chocolate muffins and protein waffles that do freeze well. Also, note that certain foods do not freeze well and will not work well in this plan. Examples of foods that I have found that do not freeze well are tofu, recipes that call for dairy, gravies, and cheesecakes.

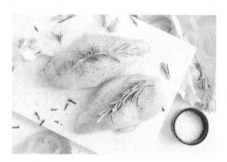

1. Pick four to six fresh vegetables to be chopped. Keep in mind that variety is required. When possible, opt for frozen vegetables to save time; however, many recipes require fresh vegetables.
2. Select four meats for the month. Half of each meat may be chopped into bite-size cubes while the other meat may be tenderized, sliced into strips, or even left whole. You may also decide to choose ground meat which can easily be used in four different ways throughout the month.
3. Source four recipes for each protein to be used in different weeks throughout the course of the month. If steaks were on sale, for example, fajitas, salsa beef, broccoli beef stir fry, and grilled steaks would be prepared.
4. Based on the recipes you plan on using, compile a list of all the ingredients you'll need. Remember to go through the freezer and pantry to see what's already there to make sure you do not buy what you already have.

The following activities will take place on prep day:

Unless they are cooked and frozen, fruits should not be prepared more than a week in advance. Breakfast is also usually something that should be done on a weekly basis, at least when you are new to meal prepping.

1. Fruits and Vegetables

- Start by preparing any vegetables that need cooking to prep – blanched zucchini for Lasagna Boats or sautéed onions for meatloaf are examples of vegetables that will need to be cooked the day of prepping.
- Vegetables that need to be cooked at the same time as meats should be chopped and added to those meats—red bell peppers for the Sweet Chili Pork, for example. Prepare other vegetables, such as zucchini spirals, and store them.
- Peel and chop all the vegetables you will need for the month, and put them in plastic freezer bags. Save time and freezer space by storing the meat and vegetables together in smaller individual bags within one large freezer bag.
- If you have a fruit that needs to be cooked before freezing, start that fruit cooking on the stovetop before moving on to the marinades and spices.

2. Marinades and Spices

- Label storage bags for all marinades and spice mixes before starting. Use smaller bags for marinades that will be frozen separate from meats and vegetables.
- Place all marinade ingredients in plastic freezer storage bags and set aside.
- Combine all spice mixes in storage bags and set aside. Get the protein ready while the spices meld together.

3. Protein

- Chop, tenderize, and weigh out one protein at a time.

Chicken should be left for last to avoid salmonella and prevent cross-contamination.

- Place all the proteins into the labeled plastic freezer storage bags with the marinades, add fresh vegetables (if using) into the bags, and seal the bags.
- Depending on when the meals will be eaten, place the sealed bags into the freezer or refrigerator.
- Clean the countertops and chopping boards thoroughly. Preferably, each protein should have its own chopping board.
- Repeat the process with all the proteins, keeping the chicken as the last protein to be prepared.

Sample Batch-Prepping Day

SAMPLE BATCH-PREPPING PLANNER			GROCERIES
PROTEINS TO PREP	**VEGETABLES TO PREP**	**FRUITS TO PREP**	
PROTEIN 1: Chicken **RECIPES:** BBQ Chicken, Orange-ginger chicken, Chicken k-bobs, Sweet and sour chicken	ginger (grated) red onions (chunked)	oranges (segmented)	4 lbs. chicken breasts 4 lbs. pork loin 4 lbs. sirloin 4 lbs. ground turkey mandarin oranges
PROTEIN 2: Pork **RECIPES:** Green chili pork stew, Sweet chili pork, Pork chops, Pork loin roast	red bell peppers (diced) onion (diced)		ginger red onion white onions red bell peppers squash or zucchini
PROTEIN 3: Beef **RECIPES:** Salsa steak, Broccoli and beef stir fry, fajitas, grilled steaks	red bell peppers (diced) onion (diced)		frozen asparagus frozen broccoli jarred mushrooms canned green chilis jarred spaghetti sauce
PROTEIN 4: Turkey **RECIPES:** Lasagna boats, Spaghetti and meatballs, Meatloaf, Chili	squash or zucchini (cored and cut in ½) red bell peppers (diced) onion (diced) zucchini (shredded)		sugar free ketchup Bragg's aminos lemon juice sweetener apple cider vinegar liquid smoke chili garlic sauce spices

1. Choose 4 proteins for variety.
2. Choose 4 recipes to go with each of the proteins you have chosen.
3. Choose vegetables to go with each recipe (no more than 6 to prep, the rest canned, jarred, or frozen).
4. Choose the fruits to eat with each meal (no more than 2 to prep, the rest canned, jarred, or frozen).
5. Create a grocery list.

For a printable version of all the sample and blank planners, scan the QR code or email us at brooksmealprepbooks@gmail.com

The purpose of the sample prep day is to show you how to work the plan with four meats you have bought in bulk. For this example, we will use chicken breasts, pork loin, sirloin, and ground turkey.

This plan may take more time than all the others, but you will have everything ready for an entire month of meals when your day ends. The batch-prepping will typically take a few hours to complete.

Planning the Day

1. Choose four proteins for variety. This sample day needs the following proteins:

- chicken breasts
- pork loin
- beef
- turkey

2. Choose four recipes to go with each type of meat. This sample day uses the following recipes:

- Barbecue chicken
- Orange-ginger chicken
- Chicken k-bobs
- Sweet and sour chicken
- Green chili pork stew
- Sweet chili pork
- Pork chops
- Pork loin roast
- Salsa steak
- Broccoli and beef stir fry
- Fajitas
- Grilled steaks
- Lasagna boats
- Spaghetti and meatballs
- Meatloaf

- Chili

3. Choose vegetables to go with each recipe. You should choose no more than six vegetables to prep and be sure the rest of the vegetables are canned, jarred, or frozen. This sample day preps the following vegetables:

- ginger
- red onions
- white or yellow onions
- red bell peppers
- zucchini or squash
- tomatillos

4. Choose no more than two fruits to prep on this day. This sample day preps the following fruits:

- mandarin oranges

5. Create a complete grocery list. Remember to go through the freezer and pantry to see what's already there to make sure you do not buy what you already have.

How the Batch-Cooking Prep Will Look

1. Start a pot of water boiling for blanching the zucchini boats.

2. Fill the sink with water and ensure the trashcan and dishwasher are empty so you can clean as you go.

3. Prepare all fruits and vegetables first:

- Peel and segment one pound of mandarin oranges.
- Cut and core four zucchini boats. Prepare ice water for blanching. Water should be boiling now, so blanch the

zucchini boats and put in freezer on lined baking sheets to freeze.

- Shred the zucchini for the meatloaf.
- Slice tomatillos and heat in microwave.
- Now dice one of the onions to sauté for the meatloaf. Start sautéing the onion while you prep the rest of the onions.
- Prepare remaining vegetables and set aside.

4. Now that all vegetables are prepared, move on to spices and marinades:

- Blend together the green chilis, tomatillos, and remaining ingredients for the sauce. Set aside in labeled gallon storage bag.
- Combine all ingredients for Salsa Steak sauce. Set aside in labeled gallon storage bag.
- Label storage bags and prepare all remaining marinades and spices.
- At this step, add vegetables to the marinades they will marinate in. The red bell peppers should be marinated with the sweet chili marinade to absorb the flavors. The peppers and onions should be marinated with the fajita seasoning.

5. Prepare all sirloin for recipes:

- Dice for Salsa Steak and Broccoli and Beef stir fry
- Tenderize, and slice for fajitas, and trim for steaks
- Use your favorite healthy steak seasoning on steaks before placing in a freezer bag.
- Add all remaining beef to marinades and sauces and place in a freezer or refrigerator.

6. Prepare all pork for recipes:

- Dice for Green Chili Stew and Sweet Chili Pork

- Trim for Pork chops, and Pork loin roast.
- Use your favorite healthy pork seasoning on pork chops before placing in a freezer bag.
- Add all remaining pork to marinades and spices and place in the freezer or refrigerator.

7. Prepare all ground turkey recipes:

- Use two pounds of ground turkey combined with spices to form meatballs and fill frozen zucchini boats
- Use one pound of ground turkey to combine with spices for chili, and use the remaining pound of turkey to combine with spices and onions for meatloaf.
- Place all turkey dishes in storage bags and move to the refrigerator or freezer.

8. Prepare all chicken recipes:

- Place chicken breasts in barbecue sauce and coat completely
- Cube chicken for k-bobs, cut into bite sized pieces for Orange-ginger chicken and Sweet and Sour chicken.
- Add all chicken to gallon bags for freezing. Chicken absorbs marinade quickly, so storing anything but the barbecue chicken in the marinade is not advised. Store marinade in a separate smaller bag with the chicken and marinate the day it will be cooked.

Although the batch-prepping plan may take longer than any other plan, it saves time by having everything prepared for an entire month. Once you are comfortable with batch-prepping, you will probably find you are able to batch-cook many foods while prepping others and have meals ready for you at the end of the day.

I've included a blank planning chart to help you get started.

BATCH-PREPPING PLANNER			GROCERIES
PROTEINS TO PREP	**VEGETABLES TO PREP**	**FRUITS TO PREP**	
PROTEIN 1: RECIPES:			
PROTEIN 2: RECIPES:			
PROTEIN 3: RECIPES:			
PROTEIN 4: RECIPES:			

1. Choose 4 proteins for variety.
2. Choose 4 recipes to go with each of the proteins you have chosen.
3. Choose vegetables to go with each recipe (no more than 6 to prep, the rest canned, jarred, or frozen).
4. Choose the fruits to eat with each meal (no more than 2 to prep, the rest canned, jarred, or frozen).
5. Create a grocery list.

For a printable version of all the sample and blank planners, scan the QR code or email us at brooksmealprepbooks@gmail.com

7

THE HYBRID MEAL-PREP PLAN

The hybrid meal-prep plan is a combination of the three plans discussed earlier. So, you prepare some of the items like you would during power hour, cook a few things for lunches and dinners like you would for the once-and-done plan, and batch prep some things for the freezer like you would for batch prepping.

This prep plan requires two and a half to three hours to put everything together, calculating six days worth of meals with three meals per day. Some items are cooked on prep day, and some items are frozen. The frozen meals can be taken from the freezer a day or two before they are needed and will be ready to quickly cook up when they are needed.

Here's how the hybrid meal-prep plan is set up:

1. Choose four to six protein recipes for the week (depending on your weight-loss program and your menu).
2. Choose one protein, and cook it on the day of meal prep. If your family doesn't like leftovers, choose this meal wisely. Foods like spaghetti, chili, meatballs, and some soups are great heated up the next day.

3. Three protein recipes should be prepared and frozen or refrigerated, ready to be cooked on the stovetop in the evening. These three recipes should include at least two different proteins for variety.

4. Prepare two more protein recipes for batch-prepping and freezing. These recipes will ideally include two different proteins that require minimal preparation and will be cooked whole, such as steak, fish, or chicken breasts.

5. Two more recipes will be breakfast recipes. Plan on cooking one the day of prepping and keep the other one raw to toss in the oven while getting ready in the morning or baking the night before.

6. Next, decide on the vegetables that will go with each protein (no more than three fresh vegetables). The rest need to be frozen or require no preparation, like cherry tomatoes and mushrooms, or come from cans and jars.

7. Decide on fresh fruits and cooked fruits for the week. Choose up to two that will require preparation, like segmented mandarin oranges, and one that can be cooked, like fresh cranberry sauce or blueberries made into syrup for protein pancakes.

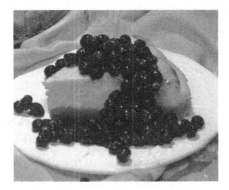

Cottage Cheesecake

Sample Hybrid Meal Prep Day

SAMPLE HYBRID MEAL PREP PLANNER			GROCERIES	
PROTEINS	**VEGETABLES**	**FRUITS**	1 lb. ground pork	
PROTEIN 1: Sausage/Protein Powder RECIPE: Mock Griddles	n/a	strawberries (cooked for jam)	1 lb. pork loin	
			2 lbs. chicken breasts	
PROTEIN 2: Eggs/Cottage Cheese RECIPE: Omelet Muffins	salsa (jarred)	blueberries (fresh)	1 lb. tilapia	
			1 lb. ground sirloin	
			pea protein powder	
PROTEIN 3: Pork RECIPE: Sweet Chili Pork	red bell pepper (prepped)	apple (whole)	egg whites	
			1% cottage cheese	
PROTEIN 4: Chicken RECIPE: Chicken K-bobs	onion + zucchini (prepped) tomatoes + mushrooms	pear (whole)	2 red bell peppers	
			1 onion	
			cherry tomatoes	
PROTEIN 5: Fish RECIPE: Italian Baked Tilapia	asparagus (frozen)	peaches (canned)	button mushrooms	
			1 zucchini	
			1 spaghetti squash	
PROTEIN 6: Ground Turkey RECIPE: Add to Spaghetti Sauce	spaghetti squash (whole)	melon (prepped)	1 jar of salsa	
			1 jar of spaghetti sauce	
PROTEIN 7 (BATCH PREP): Beef RECIPE: Hamburger Patties	onions or bell peppers (diced for patties)	n/a	canned peaches	
			strawberries	
			melon	
PROTEIN 8 (BATCH PREP): Chicken RECIPE: Orange-Ginger Chicken	grated ginger (prepped)	mandarin oranges (prepped)	blueberries	
			apples	
			pears	
1. Choose 6 proteins for variety to cook on prep day and 2 more to batch prep for later cooking.			mandarin oranges	
2. Choose recipes to go with the proteins you have chosen.				
3. Choose vegetables to go with each recipe (no more than 4 to prep, the rest canned, jarred, or frozen).				
4. Choose the fruits to eat with each meal (no more than 3 to prep, the rest canned, jarred, or frozen).				
5. Create a grocery list.				

For a printable version of all the sample and blank planners, scan the QR code or email us at brooksmealprepbooks@gmail.com

The purpose of this sample is to show you how to implement the hybrid meal-prep plan with six proteins. If you are on intermittent fasting, omit two proteins and use only four. The proteins for this sample prep day are MockGriddles, oven-baked omelet muffins, sweet chili pork, chicken k-bobs, Italian baked tilapia, Italian turkey sausage, orange ginger chicken, and hamburgers.

This plan takes less than 3 hours if you follow these guidelines:

- Prep four dinner proteins with marinades that may be frozen or can stay raw until the evening they will be eaten (sweet chili pork, chicken k-bobs, Italian baked tilapia, and orange ginger chicken). The marinades for the chicken and fish should be placed in a storage bag separate from the meat until ready to marinate, as fish and chicken take on too much marinade flavor to be frozen in the marinade. Chicken can be marinated for up to 24 hours, and fish should only be marinated for 30 minutes.

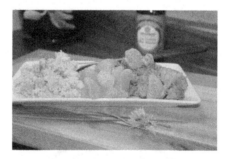

Orange Ginger Chicken

- Batch prep two dinner proteins to be used this week and in future weeks (Italian turkey sausage and hamburger patties), and fully cook two meals (MockGriddles with breakfast sausage and Italian turkey sausage with spaghetti squash).
- When choosing recipes, find ones that use the same types of vegetables. Choosing more than four types of vegetables to prep will add a lot of time to the meal prep.

- Prepare the following vegetables: onions prepared in two ways (diced and chopped), zucchini, grated ginger, and red bell peppers.
- The other vegetables should be whole, frozen, or jarred—cherry tomatoes, button mushrooms, jarred salsa and spaghetti sauce, and frozen asparagus for this sample plan.
- Choose no more than three fruits that need to be prepped: cooked strawberries, chopped melon, and segmented mandarin oranges for this sample plan.
- The other fruits will be added fresh and eaten whole. You can get these canned, but these usually have added ingredients that will just make you hungrier! Peeling your own oranges, for example, is worth the extra effort—that way you avoid additives.

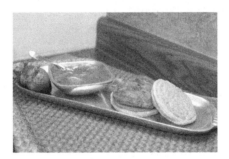

MockGriddles

How the Day Will Look:

1. Preheat your oven to 350 degrees and adjust recipe times to accommodate one temperature. If a recipe calls for 300 degrees, you will need to cook it longer. Conversely, if a recipe calls for 400 degrees, you will cook it for less time. I have found that using one oven temperature for everything will save loads of time and the dishes will turn out just fine.

2. Fill the sink with soapy water and empty the trashcan and dishwasher. Be sure you have all the ingredients and tools you need.

3. Place the vegetables that will be cooked whole (spaghetti squash) on a foil-lined cookie sheet, and put them into the oven to start roasting.

4. Create the four marinades, and set aside.

- sweet chili pork marinade
- chicken k-bob marinade
- Italian fish marinade
- orange ginger chicken marinade

5. Create the spice mixtures, and set aside.

- Italian sausage spices
- breakfast sausage spices
- any desired spices for hamburgers

6. Prepare all vegetables and all fruits before starting on the meat.

- slice and dice onions
- slice red bell peppers
- rinse cherry tomatoes
- wipe down mushrooms
- peel and segment mandarin oranges
- start simmering strawberries for jam on MockGriddles

7. Start with the meal you will be cooking today.

- In a large bowl, mix the turkey with the Italian seasoning, and mix well.
- Place in a large nonstick frying pan, and start cooking over medium heat, watching closely while you work on the next step.

8. Prepare all other meats.

- Add hamburger meat to seasoning, add onions, and make patties. Then put the patties into the freezer. The onions will keep the patties from drying out while frozen. If you don't like onions, replace them with any type of pepper, shredded squash, or even shredded carrots.
- Add lean ground pork to breakfast sausage spices, and make patties. Set aside to cook when the Italian turkey sausage is finished cooking.
- Prepare the pork for the sweet chili pork recipe, cut it into pieces, and add to the marinade with onions and red bell peppers. Place in the freezer.
- The tilapia should not be frozen in the same bag as the marinade because the marinade will overpower the fish. So, freeze them in separate bags.
- Place chicken breasts and mandarin oranges into a freezer bag, and freeze. Do not freeze with the marinade. The marinade should be frozen in a separate bag and only combined with the chicken the night before it will be cooked. Oranges will lose their sweetness within about a week of freezing, so use them this week. The oranges will be added toward the end of cooking but should be prepped ahead of time.
- Chop up chicken for k-bobs. Don't freeze with the marinade. The marinade should be frozen in a separate bag and only combined with the chicken the night before it will be cooked. These will be assembled before cooking.

9. Finish the dinner recipe that is cooked for consumption today - spaghetti and meat sauce.

- Transfer the cooked Italian turkey sausage to a pot, add your favorite marinara sauce, and simmer for about a half hour. Let cool.

10. Now, cook the breakfasts.

- Start by washing out the large frying pan, and cook pork sausage patties on medium while preparing the MockGriddle muffin mixture.
- Mix ingredients for MockGriddle muffins, and set aside until the sausage patties are done.
- Mix all the ingredients for the omelet muffins, and separate into equal-size ramekins to bake when ready to eat.
- Remove sausage from the pan, and start cooking the MockGriddle muffins.

11. Remove the spaghetti squash from the oven. Cut it open to let it cool down while you clean up.

12. While watching the MockGriddle muffins and letting the squash cool, clean the entire kitchen. Keep a close eye on the MockGriddle muffins so they don't burn.

13. After the kitchen is cleaned, bag up the MockGriddles for breakfast, scoop the spaghetti squash into a container, and pour cooled spaghetti sauce into a container (or leave it in the same pot it simmered in if you will be using it soon).

This plan takes a lot of coordinating and planning, but the benefits of not only having your meals prepared, but other ingredients prepped and frozen for a later date make the plan worth the upfront planning time.

I've included a blank planning chart to help you get started.

HYBRID MEAL PREP PLANNER			GROCERIES	
PROTEINS	**VEGETABLES**	**FRUITS**		
PROTEIN 1: RECIPE:				
PROTEIN 2: RECIPE:				
PROTEIN 3: RECIPE:				
PROTEIN 4: RECIPE:				
PROTEIN 5: RECIPE:				
PROTEIN 6: RECIPE:				
PROTEIN 7 (BATCH PREP): RECIPE:				
PROTEIN 8 (BATCH PREP): RECIPE:				

1. Choose 6 proteins for variety to cook on prep day and 2 more to batch prep for later cooking.
2. Choose recipes to go with the proteins you have chosen.
3. Choose vegetables to go with each recipe (no more than 4 to prep, the rest canned, jarred, or frozen).
4. Choose the fruits to eat with each meal (no more than 3 to prep, the rest canned, jarred, or frozen).
5. Create a grocery list.

For a printable version of all the sample and blank planners, scan the QR code or email us at brooksmealprepbooks@gmail.com

8

WHAT I DID FOR WEIGHT LOSS AND HOW I KEEP THE WEIGHT OFF

Before discussing how I lost the weight, please let me emphasize that I had help from a nutritionist, a doctor, and knowledgeable physical therapists. They all helped me learn to listen to my own body in order to make changes as needed. I strongly encourage you seek the advice of a nutritionist for a personalized plan, and I also encourage you speak with your primary doctor to determine a plan that is safe for you. I am including what worked for me personally not as a guideline for your own journey, but as a personal account of my own journey.

Different plans work for different people and lifestyles. Through the years, I've tried many plans to lose weight, but intermittent fasting has worked best for my body. When I wanted to lose weight, I restricted myself to an 8-hour eating window and only two meals. Now that I'm happy with my weight and my health, I restrict myself to a 10-hour eating window with three meals. The benefits of this are numerous, so I stick with it. Meal prepping is what helps me stick to this plan!

Here are my before and after pictures for context. In the first picture I weighed 162 pounds, and in the second I weighed 125 pounds. This weight loss occurred over a 5 month span.

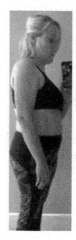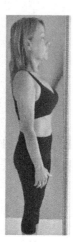

The reasons I chose this plan are as follows:

- An 8-hour restricted-eating window has been shown to help stabilize hormones and chronic inflammation. I've suffered from hormonal irregularities and chronic inflammation for years. Intermittent fasting helps me feel much better and more in control of what my body is doing, including regulating thyroid problems, which I've had for several years.
- I found studies that supported the concept of intermittent fasting like one study that showed, intermittent fasting helped women lose weight by lowering body fat, and regulating menstruation, reduced chronic inflammation, and improved insulin resistance (Li et al., 2021). I struggled in all these areas, so this was the study that convinced me to try intermittent fasting.
- A Keto diet with intermittent fasting made me feel better, but it didn't help me lose weight. I felt like I had enough body fat for my brain and body to use, and I didn't feel better when I added more fats to my diet. I suspected I should reduce the

amount of fat I ate, and I was right. I also felt like I needed fruit, and I was right again. Sometimes you just have to listen to your body. So I did a little more research, sought the help of a nutritionist and switched from Keto to Paleo. I think my body needs fruit to keep sugar cravings at bay, and I feel better if I have only a couple of tablespoons of fat at a meal.

- One of the studies I found talked about a peptide called GLP-1 and another peptide called GIP. They are both glucose peptides, and the study showed that after switching to the Paleo diet, the levels of both peptides went up. Why that is important is that higher levels of these peptides correlate with a lower risk of type 2 diabetes and can help control cravings. Helping with cravings along with a family history of diabetes were the primary reasons I decided to try the Paleo diet.

So, I do a combination of intermittent fasting and Paleo-ish eating, with a lot of intuition thrown in. It took a few months of food journaling to see my patterns and figure out what my body likes and doesn't like, what helps me lose weight the most, and what makes me feel best. I highly recommend food journaling so you can go back to see which foods affect you and in what ways.

I also eat a lot of protein. I was temporarily in a wheelchair after a surgical complication, was later unable to walk without a walker, and then used a cane for months. What I learned in physical therapy is this: Protein is king, and electrolytes are queen. If you feel weak or your muscles shake when you try to lift something, you may need more protein. If you feel weak and light-headed, you may need electrolytes and more fluids in general. You may want to add a high-quality sugar-free electrolyte to your daily routine. I find that I get plenty of electrolytes by putting lemon or lime juice with a pinch of pink salt in my water (no more than 1/4 teaspoon of salt for the entire day).

Here's how my plan works:

- I find that drinking fennel tea helps calm my hunger and desire to snack, so I drink a lot of that. Fennel is said to have many benefits, such as regulating menstrual periods, boosting immunity, and possibly improving brain function.
- If I'm not exercising, I do intermittent fasting, eat low-fat foods, and eat only two meals a day. I try to eat only during the one 8-hour window per day, but sometimes it ends up being a 10-hour window because life happens. I don't do 8-hour intermittent fasting or low-fat food for more than 6 weeks at a time, because it seems to stress out my body.
- To lose the weight, I did 6 weeks of intermittent fasting followed by 6 weeks of three meals a day and then went back to fasting. Once I lost all the weight I wanted to lose (I lost about 6 pounds a month), I went back to three meals a day and added no more than 2 tablespoons of fat per meal.
- I rotate foods (I discussed how this affects weight loss in a previous chapter). If I eat a specific kind of food, I wait 48 hours to eat that food again, except for peppers, mushrooms, and greens like lettuce, spinach, kale, cucumbers, and celery.
- I eat celery or cucumber or even low-sodium pickles between meals if I get really hungry.

If you want to try it out, first, figure out how much protein your body requires every day. As covered in Chapter 2, 0.36 grams per pound of body weight is the minimum recommended to maintain muscle. So, for a 150-pound person, this would translate to 54 grams of protein. There are about 7 grams of protein in an ounce of cooked meat, so this would mean a person who weighs 150 pounds would need to consume a minimum of 8 ounces of meat for the day. If more protein is needed, extra can easily be added with healthy options like 1% cottage cheese or fat-free plain Greek yogurt in place of sour cream. Some recipes can even be adapted with vegan substitutions like tofu.

Each weight-loss-cycle meal is made up like this:

- Determine your protein needs. Use the correct ounces of very lean protein (lower-fat turkey or chicken meat like white meat or no lower than 93% hamburger (sirloin is the only steak I eat now), the highest-percent lean ground pork you can find, pork loin, uncured turkey bacon, cod or tilapia, tofu, 1% cottage cheese, egg whites, etc.).
- To make things simple and ensure I'm getting enough fruit, I just match the ounces of fruit to my ounces of protein. If I really want starch, I'll eat 50 calories' worth of bread, tortillas, rice, and so forth in place of fruit. I don't eat both at the same time. The fruit has many more nutrients, and I feel better eating the fruit, so I don't replace fruit with starch more than a couple of times a week. Focus on low-glycemic, low-fat fruit (no pineapple, no grapes, no coconut, no bananas, etc.).
- I match my ounces of vegetables to my ounces of protein and add more of those vegetables, like lettuce, peppers, onions, and celery, that I don't rotate if I want to feel fuller. Focus on non-starchy low-fat vegetables (no potatoes, no corn, no avocados, etc.).
- During my meals, I eat as much onion, peppers, celery, lettuce, or cucumber as I need in order to stay full between meals. I avoid snacking between meals. That's an important part of intermittent fasting. It helps your hormones work better so you will lose weight more easily. If you absolutely must snack, choose only low-sodium pickles, cucumber, lettuce, celery, or peppers. If any of these disagree with your body, do something different until the next meal.
- I cook everything in a broth. I don't use oils or butter for cooking. I can always add fats afterward in a much more controlled way. If I absolutely must for a certain pot or pan, I use the smallest amount of spray oil I can get by with.

I've found that when I don't exercise, I can get by with 8 ounces of lean protein for the day. It's just different for everyone. When I am exercising, I seem to need 10–12 ounces to keep from feeling starved. I try not to worry if I feel hungry on intermittent fasting, but I don't let myself feel starved.

- When I am exercising, I do everything the same as above, but I eat three meals a day. You don't have to add vegetables to breakfast, but I find it gives me more energy and more fiber if I do, so I feel better and less hungry. I'll add cauliflower or pumpkin to a protein shake or lots of veggies to an egg white omelet.

When I just need a break and I'm exercising, this is what I do to maintain my weight:

- I eat three meals a day but add no more than 2 tablespoons of fat or half an avocado to lunch and dinner. I do not add fat to my breakfast. I feel like it bogs me down, and it seems to make me gain weight.
- If I gain more than a few pounds, I reduce my fat a little.

Here are some ways I make this work for my family:

- The family eats whatever they want for breakfast and lunch, and I prepare what I need in advance.
- When they eat pasta, I eat a pasta substitute made from hearts of palm, or I eat spaghetti squash, zucchini squash spirals, or mashed or riced cauliflower.
- The only dairy I eat is 1% cottage cheese. My family can add other cheeses, like parmesan or cheddar, to foods like fajitas and burgers.
- When my family eats tortillas, I usually put whatever they are putting into a tortilla on top of a salad.

- If they are eating bread, I will usually use iceberg lettuce instead.
- If the family is eating potatoes, I will make myself a half of a small sweet potato in place of my fruit for that meal.
- I use plain, nonfat Greek yogurt instead of sour cream.
- I prepare most of my dinner meals to be cooked when I get home from work and use the leftovers for my lunches. That way everyone gets a fresh meal in the evening.
- Sometimes we all eat something different. And sometimes I just eat what they are eating. Especially if it's pizza!

I've tried to create recipes they all love, so it's been pretty easy to make it work.

How Meal Prepping Helped Me

Meal prepping was the most important factor in successfully losing weight because it helped me stay on track and learn to listen to the needs of my body. On the weeks I didn't meal prep, I would find myself eating more than my body needed or even grabbing a quick takeout meal for lunch that would sabotage all my hard work. This realization kept me committed to learning to enjoy meal prepping.

When I first started meal prepping I would spend six or seven hours on the weekend just crying and cussing in the kitchen. You see, I don't like to cook, I never have. I would wake up early on a Saturday and chaotically cook every single thing I was going to eat that week. The amount of work this took was enough to help keep me committed to my weight loss plan. This was a frustrating time for me, but I learned so much from the experience.

I would start by creating a menu for the week that included rotation of foods, and plan my prep and grocery shopping around the menu. This weekly menu along with a food journal allowed me to go back and find foods that were interfering with my goals. I personally found that tomatoes, which are one of my favorite foods, cause me pain, inflammation, and weight gain. This was the most shocking and possibly the most helpful discovery of meal prepping for me.

I eventually learned little meal prepping hacks like that prepping all the fruits and vegetables in my plan was taking a lot of precious time and if I limited those and opted for frozen, jarred, or caned when possible I would finish my prep faster. Another thing I learned was that waiting for the oven temperature to change from recipe to recipe took much too long, and I learned to adapt my recipes around one oven temperature. Little changes like these saved me hours in the kitchen, making it easier for me to continue meal prepping.

The more I meal prepped and journaled, the more I was able to notice foods that triggered me. I realized that excitotoxins in certain seasonings left me starved before the next meal, and I learned how to create my own seasonings. I noticed that fish didn't fill me up for long and I needed to eat a large salad with extra vegetables on fish nights. I noticed so many ways different foods affected me that I was able to adjust my meals to meet the needs of my body and my health began to improve. With my health improving, the weight seemed to come off easier, and my energy also improved. As time passed, I was able to intuitively sense what my body needed without looking back and comparing my food journal to my menu.

Had it not been for planning and prepping my meals, I would not have learned to listen to the needs of my body. I am a much healthier, energetic, and thinner person today because of what meal prepping taught me.

9

MINDSET FOR SUCCESS

Arguably the most important aspect of any success in life is mindset. Having a positive outlook and believing you can reach the goals you've set out to accomplish are both key to all success. In order to be successful at meal prepping and weight loss, it it important to have a positive outlook and an expectation of great success. This attitude will get you through the bumps in the road and yes, there will be bumps in the road.

Let's talk about some ways we can adopt a positive mindset about change.

- **Know your why**

A very important aspect of motivating yourself to keep going when things aren't turning out the way you want is having a clear understanding of why you want to keep going. For me, this was very personal. I had just gotten out of a wheelchair and was still having difficulty walking. I'd had three doctors tell me that losing 20 pounds would help me walk unassisted again. I desperately wanted to walk without a walker or a cane, and that was my why. At first, I remember thinking that I couldn't even walk for exercise, so losing weight seemed impossible. I had to change my mindset.

Knowing why you want this change is so important. You need to be clear on why it is important to you and no-one else. This should be something personal to you, or it isn't going to have the power behind it to get you through the rough times. Learning a new way of preparing meals and learning to cook in healthier ways can be a challenge at times. Being clear about your why will help you remember that overcoming any challenge is worth it in the long run.

Take a while to reflect on your why. Write it down and keep it close to you so you can be reminded of your reason or reasons frequently. This is an important and proven aspect of personal success. There are several videos and articles online to help you with your why if you are still struggling to find the words.

- **Believe in yourself**

Most of us have friends and family who think we are wonderful and strong, and believe in our ability to accomplish anything. Having a strong support group is helpful, but it is nothing compared to belief in ourselves.

To illustrate the long term challenges of weight loss, researchers of a two year study of weight loss maintenance found that when participants perceived their new healthy life style and routine as sustainable and had the mindset that they could maintain the weight loss, they kept the weight off. Simply put, they believed in themselves. The participants with weight gain at the end of the study were shown to have the mindset of not being able to stick to a plan during times of emotional stress. Simply put, they did not believe in themselves.

Seeing meal prepping as a way of life that you are able to maintain long term, no matter your current life circumstances could be an important factor in reaching and maintaining your goals. Fostering belief in yourself isn't always easy, but it can be done. Think back to your accomplishments of the past. You've done hard things, completed hard tasks, and won victories no matter how small. Use those as a solid foundation on which to build your self belief.

Set small goals for yourself daily and check those off a list as you accomplish each goal. This will train your brain to think of yourself as a winner who can accomplish bigger things. Don't let negative self-talk creep into your mind - we will discuss this further in a bit.

- **Don't make excuses**

Admitting that you need to change your mindset may be the most difficult part of changing your mindset. If you aren't happy with your current situation however, there's a strong possibility that your mindset needs shifting.

If you find yourself saying you can't do something because...it doesn't matter the because, then you are making excuses. Find a work around. Find a solution. There are always solutions to problems.

I can't eat healthy because my family won't eat healthy is a common excuse. There are solutions. You may need to eat something completely different from what your family eats, or you may need to find ways to turn their favorite recipes into more healthy meals. You may also need to make substitutions. Keep the mindset that you can and will find a solution rather than the mindset of excuses.

We can make excuses for why we can't do so many things, but there is usually a good workaround that will enable us to accomplish the goals we've set for ourselves. Making excuses or blaming others only sets our minds up to fail. If failure is not what you desire, but you would rather have success, start taking matters into your own hands instead of making excuses. Looking past the reasons we can't accomplish a goal can be the hardest part of becoming successful, but it's worth all the effort.

- **Meditate and Visualize**

So, how can you change your mind to feel positive and better able to achieve your goals? Mindset can be changed by consistently feeding your mind with positive thoughts of success.

Meditation and visualization have been shown to help many people reach their goals. In 2014 researchers reviewed fourteen studies and found that through meditation the study participants decreased binge eating, emotional eating, and weight gain. Their minds, not their willpower changed their actions!

Visualizing yourself succeeding at your goal is a powerful meditative tool that seems to help the subconscious embrace the idea that you can meet your goals. Imagine yourself five or ten years from now if you don't change a thing. You're still eating foods that don't agree with your, and you've gained weight. Are you happier? Are you healthier? How do you feel? Then, imagine yourself five or ten years from now when you have made healthy changes. You've learned how to meal prep. You've lost weight and become more active. How are you feeling now? Are you happier? Are you healthier? Of course you are. These are powerful thoughts and images that can change your life for the better.

There are many guided visualization and meditation videos available on the internet that can help you learn these techniques.

- **Develop a mindset of change**

Another way to change your mindset is to simply begin embracing change. This mindset of change adopts the idea that we are not stuck being the way we are, but that we can change. Believing that you can get better at managing your stress without food, believing that you can become faster at meal prepping, and believing that you can become better at cooking healthier meals are all important beliefs that will get you through even the toughest times.

There are two types of mindset: the stuck mindset and the mind that is open to change. A person with a stuck mindset believes they are not capable of change. A person with a stuck mindset would think that they've tried to lose weight before and it didn't work, so there is no use. A person with a mindset of change believes they can change over time. The person with the mindset of change would believe that they learn from their failures and would let those failures help them to be successful the next time they face the same sort of obstacle.

To adopt the mindset of change, remind yourself that a setback doesn't define you. If you slip up in any way, do not accept that as just who you are. Refocus on your goals, and move on towards change.

Another aspect of the mindset of change is understanding that not everything will change at once. Maybe it hasn't happened yet, but believing that it can and will happen is the best mindset to have. Don't let yourself get discouraged because something is taking a while; keep moving towards the change you want.

Allowing yourself to accept the change and grieve what is changing can also be beneficial. When I started on my journey back to health, I grieved food. I missed my favorite comfort foods, and I had to allow myself to let go of those things because in the long run they weren't actually bringing me comfort. Sometimes it just helps if we allow ourselves to let go of the past.

Switching your beliefs to a mindset of change could powerfully impact your success at both meal prepping and weight loss.

- **Positive self-talk.**

An aspect many successful people, including professional athletes use to foster success is positive self-talk. You can view self talking NFL players online to see this in action. Many of us go through our day with self-talk in the background of our minds. This is called your internal dialogue, and it's important that you control this dialogue in order to be successful. When this talk is negative, when you say to yourself that you can't do something, you are setting yourself up to fail.

A study in 2020 showed that people who engaged in positive self-talk had developed better strategies for coping with anxiety and mental stress. Another 2019 study looked at how positive self-talk before students gave a speech reduced their anxiety. These studies show that if you struggle with stress eating, the practice of self talk could be a helpful tool for handling stress, which in turn could help you reach your weight loss goals.

The next time you find yourself thinking you can't do something, start positive self-talk. Remind yourself how much you've already accomplished, how strong you are, and how you are not a quitter. Cheer yourself on, and watch as your mindset changes.

When I began meal prepping, I found that I didn't enjoy the new healthier foods as much as I'd enjoyed the old foods that were previously making me unhealthy and overweight. I had to do a lot of positive self-talk during those times when I literally grieved over the loss of the foods I loved. That positive self-talk got me through the sugar withdrawals, the withdrawals from the chemicals in the processed foods I'd been eating, and got me to a much better place. It's interesting to note that those favorite foods no longer taste incredible like I remembered. It was not only my mindset, but my tastebuds that changed.

- **Keep a Journal**

Write to yourself. This doesn't have to be a food journal, but food journaling can be a very helpful tool. Journaling about your struggles can relieve some of the stress related to learning new things and reaching for new goals. Journaling about your successes can help you feel stronger the next time you face a challenge. You may just find that journaling even helps you find answers to questions you might have.

Journaling can help change your mindset by helping you see why you think a certain way. Knowing why, can help you change those thoughts, if the thoughts need to be more positive. Journaling for just five minutes a day can make a big difference in shifting your mindset to be more positive because it can help you see mistakes and failures in new ways.

Start journaling by asking yourself questions like "How do I feel about eating at the party this weekend?", or "What good eating choices did I make yesterday?" Taking the time to think about upcoming temptations and celebrate successes will gradually shift your mindset to automatically knowing that you can handle anything that comes your way.

- **Notice the positive**

When you start getting bogged down with feelings of overwhelm or failure, take time to pause and appreciate. Try to focus on three positive things about yourself or your environment. This overrides the negative and retrains your brain to be more positive over time.

Stop, take a deep breath and look around you. Think back to yesterday. What went well? Did you cook a new recipe you enjoyed? Think about things you have to look forward to in the future. Do you have something exciting to look forward to? Think about this very moment. What is good right now? Just take the time to notice the good, and gradually your mind will start finding the positive in even the most mundane daily items and experiences. Before you know it, you will be more optimistic, and that positive attitude will help you succeed.

- **Understand that willpower may not be enough**

Sometimes we think if we try hard enough we will meet the goals we've set for ourselves. This may be true in many areas, but when it comes to weight loss, for most of us, willpower is not enough.

Maybe you are doing a great job sticking to your weight loss plan and you have a wedding to attend. You know your willpower is strong and you're going to stay away from the wedding cake and champagne. But, your willpower is limited, you only have so much in your tank to get you through the day. If you don't have a good plan, you may find that you've used up all your willpower on your road trip to the wedding, and there just isn't any left by the time you get there.

Realizing that we need a plan to help us use less willpower throughout the day will help. You may need to eat healthy fruits to keep your sugar cravings at bay before an event. You may need to promise yourself a piece of healthy homemade cheesecake when you get home, or you may just need to plan on a little sliver of something or a little sip of something and move on.

Don't beat yourself up when your willpower isn't enough. Blaming yourself does not foster a good mindset. Try to come up with a better plan for the next time you are faced with the same or similar challenge and get stronger from the experience.

- **Create specific goals**

How can you get to where you're going if you don't know where you are going? You wouldn't go on a trip without knowing exactly where you were going and approximately how long it would take you to reach your destination. You would also have a plan to get to your destination wouldn't you? You can do the same thing with weight loss and other goals.

Start by deciding on where you are going and how long you expect to take to reach your destination, for example what weight you will be by the end of the month. Determine what you will do to reach your goal, for example what meals or snacks you will prepare ahead of time to help with temptations. Finally, write this all down to remind yourself often of what you are going to achieve and how it will be achieved.

I find it helpful to read my plan out loud in the morning when I get out of bed and in the evening when I am getting into bed.

- **Start small**

You don't have to change everything all at once. Remember, a positive mindset has a lot to do with accepting change, but change can take time. When it comes to weight loss and meal prepping, you can start with one meal. Choose breakfast, lunch, or dinner and make it healthier. This can easily be incorporated into your life using the power hour plan. Once you have mastered one meal, you can move on to the others when you are ready, and eventually you will be eating a healthy diet. Remember, small changes are still changes that can make a big impact.

No matter how small you start, just get started. Change those negatives into positives. Changing your mindset is like watering a plant. Give the mind what it needs and what it can tolerate a little at a time and watch it grow.

10

TIPS AND TRICKS FOR EFFICIENT MEAL PREP

S logging away in the kitchen for hours is not everyone's idea of fun, but we all have to eat. Knowing a few tricks for efficient meal prep will have you in and out of the kitchen in no time.

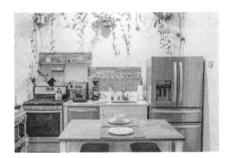

Cooking Tips

- A piece of well-done, lean meat, be it beef, chicken, pork, or lamb, will shrink to around 66% of its original raw weight.
- Cooked frozen vegetables shrink to approximately 66% of their original raw weight, and fresh vegetables will shrink to about 75% of their original weight.

- By using a meat thermometer, you will avoid overcooking or undercooking all types of meats, from steaks to chicken breasts.
- To save time, bake foods that require the same temperature together.

Freezer-Storage Tips

Raw meat, poultry, and fish

- Place a damp cotton ball in the freezer bag to keep frozen meat, such as chicken breasts or pork loin, from drying out in the freezer.
- Before freezing patties, like sausage or hamburger patties, mix in chopped onions, jalapeños, or other wet vegetables. This will keep them from drying up.
- Defrost chicken, meat, and fish in the refrigerator. Make sure it's thoroughly defrosted before cooking it.

Stews, broths, and soups

- Because you are not going to use that entire gallon of broth all at once, divide your batch into smaller batches so you can grab only what you need for a recipe without having to defrost an entire frozen block.
- You can freeze finished soups and stews for up to 2 months; if you keep them frozen longer, you risk having that unpleasant freezer burn taste. Also, the flavors start to fade at around 2 months. Broths can be frozen a bit longer.
- The best way to thaw stews and soups is slowly; this ensures the food stays at a safe temperature (40 °F) and allows it to thaw evenly. So, defrost stews and soups in the refrigerator. If time is the enemy, put your freezer bag in a bowl, and run cool water over it. Never defrost in hot water—this creates fertile ground for bacteria to grow.

Casseroles

- Line your casserole dish with aluminum foil, fill it with your ingredients, then bake your casserole and freeze it. Lift the frozen casserole out of the dish whole, tightly wrap it up, and store it in a freezer bag.
- The best way to thaw casseroles is in the fridge; this ensures the food stays at a safe temperature (40 °F) and allows it to thaw evenly.

Herbs and vegetables

- After washing and chopping herbs, preserve them by freezing them in ice cube trays filled with water. Once frozen, put the cubes in a freezer bag, and return them to the freezer.
- If you want vegetables such as green beans to keep their snap and zucchinis to keep their texture, blanch them before freezing. Vegetables such as tomatoes, squash, and okra soften when cooked and can be frozen raw in a freezer bag.
- Herbs can be frozen for 1 or 2 months and vegetables for between 2 and 3 months. Herbs and vegetables should be defrosted in the fridge if you want them defrosted, but you don't even need to defrost them—just throw them in the pot or pan, and cook.

Fruit

- If you want your fruit to keep its shape—say you want to use those strawberries in sugar free jam, for example—spread individual berries on a baking sheet and freeze them. When they are frozen hard, transfer them into a freezer bag. This can also work with fruit slices or cubes. Avocados can also be frozen. Once sliced and frozen, they are ready for guacamole.
- Fruit will last between 2 and 3 months in the freezer.
- Thaw fruit on the countertop or in the fridge. Berries and

sliced fruit have a high sugar content and therefore will take as little as 30 minutes to defrost. If you're making smoothies, you can also just toss them into a blender.

Sauces and condiments

- Freeze sauces and condiments in ice cube trays, and transfer them into freezer bags once frozen. If the ice cube method is not convenient for you, opt for smaller snack-size freezer bags.
- Water based sauces and condiments can be frozen for up to 4 months. Condiments like aioli, mayonnaise, and vinaigrette cannot be frozen. Because they are emulsified oil-based condiments, they will split when frozen, and the product will change.

General Freezing Tips

- Using ordinary zipper freezer bags without the slider is a better alternative, as it allows you to get the most air out of the bag. If the food is not well sealed, moisture will leak to other portions of the bag, causing the food to dry out.
- To effortlessly remove the air from a single freezer bag, make a small gap in the center, and suck the air out before swiftly sealing the bag. Alternately, half fill a big bucket or sink with water for sealing numerous freezer bags at once. Leave a tiny gap at the top of the bag, and immerse the bags in water, making sure water doesn't get into the bag. The air will be pushed out when you press down on the bag.
- Things should be frozen flat and stacked. Whether it's soups, stews, or ground beef, the flatter and broader you can get them, the faster they'll freeze and thaw, which saves time.
- To avoid freezer burn, allow food to cool before putting it in the freezer, but never leave items out to cool for more than 2

hours. Also, this speeds up freezing, and the food will retain its flavor, color, and texture.

- To get food frozen as rapidly as possible, don't freeze more than 4 quarts at a time, and avoid freezing anything thicker than 3 inches in height.
- The faster food freezes, the better the quality when thawed. Place containers in a single layer to enable adequate space for air to circulate around them and allow food to freeze quickly. Take care not to overcrowd the freezer. Food frozen slowly develops ice crystals, which can cause the meal to become mushy. Most prepared foods may be frozen for 2–3 months. You may also use a freezer thermometer to ensure that the temperature of your frozen food remains at 0 °F.
- If the food within a container does not reach the top, place a sheet of waxed paper in direct contact with the food before sealing to help avoid freezer burn.
- Food should always be labeled and dated. Use the first-in, first-out approach; this will help minimize food waste.
- Defrost food in the refrigerator or microwave. To avoid contamination, never thaw food at room temperature.

Refrigerated Fruit and Vegetable Storage

- Fruit that is stored in glass containers such as mason jars will survive up to three times as long.
- To keep fresh-washed greens fresher for longer, store them in plastic or glass containers lined with paper towels.
- Wrapping low-acid vegetables like celery, onions, and carrots in foil can keep them fresher for longer.
- To keep sliced apples, avocados, pears, and other fruit from turning brown, store them in water with a few drops of lemon juice or apple cider vinegar.

Additional Tips

- When possible, use containers that can go from the freezer to the oven.
- Cast-iron pans can be used from stove top to oven.
- Debone your store-bought rotisserie chicken while it's still hot, as the meat will be easier to pull off; once it cools down, it won't come off the bones as easily.
- Instead of plates, use cheap coffee filters as containers for food that has been chopped and needs to be set aside for weighing or is waiting to be cooked, such as onions, bell peppers, or squash. This works well for dry vegetables and cuts down on time spent washing dishes.
- Use scissors or kitchen shears to quickly cut meat without a knife.
- Use a pizza slicer to quickly mince fresh herbs.

On a final note, try not to refreeze thawed food. Even though food that has been properly frozen and thawed can be refrozen without concern of bacterial contamination, it is not recommended. The processes of freezing, defrosting, and refreezing damage the texture, taste, and color of many foods, making them less appealing.

11

RECIPES

These are many of the recipes I meal prepped to help me take off the weight and regain my health. There are two types of recipes: hands-off and hands-on. Remember when you are meal prepping for the week, it's best to make no more than half the recipes hands-on.

Let's talk about ingredients:

These recipes all call for what I consider to be lean proteins. For my weight loss I used many simplified ideas, deciding on what I considered to be a leaner fat content for a food was no different. I determined whether a protein was leaner based on how its fat content compared to that of a chicken breast, and I then tried to get as close to that amount of fat as I could when I chose cuts of meat. As I stated in an earlier chapter, I like to add in my fats like nuts, oils, or avocado in a controlled way after my food is cooked.

I am in no way saying that fats are inherently bad, in fact we need fats for proper health. However, too much of anything can cause troubles, and having more control of what could cause us trouble is always helpful.

Here's a helpful approximate comparison of proteins based on data from the USDA database:

Chicken Breast: 4 oz. = 4 grams of fat

Chicken Thigh: 4 oz. = 10 grams of fat

Pork Loin: 4 oz. = 7 grams of fat

Pork Chop: 4 oz. = 16 grams of fat

Sirloin: 4 oz. = 13 grams of fat

Ribeye: 4 oz. = 25 grams of fat

93% Ground Beef: 4 oz. = 8 grams of fat

83% Ground Beef: 4 oz. = 22 grams of fat

1% Cottage Cheese: 4 oz = 1 gram of fat

4% Cottage Cheese: 4 oz. = 5 grams of fat

Egg Whites: 4 oz. = 0.3 grams of fat

Eggs: 4oz. = 11 grams of fat

The sautéed foods are meant to be cooked in broth, not butter or oil, while the baked dishes are meant to be baked using the minimum amount of cooking spray possible. If your weight loss program allows fats, it's easy to add those later in controlled amounts.

When a recipe calls for a pre-packaged ingredient, say ketchup or spaghetti sauce, the intent is that you will choose a very healthy brand with no excitotoxins or chemically altered sweeteners. Remember, excitotoxins are meant to trick your brain into eating more than you planned.

If Greek yogurt is called for, this is referring to nonfat, unflavored Greek yogurt. If cottage cheese is called for, this means using 1% cottage cheese.

Sea salt is full of minerals your body needs, so when I use salt in a recipe that is what I use. Salt is always optional. If you choose not to use salt, try adding more of the other spices in the recipe to add to the flavor.

Sugar substitutes are a great way to satisfy a sweet tooth. I have made these recipes with either monkfruit drops or a granulated monkfruit with erythritol blend. Other naturally derived sugar substitutes that shouldn't spike blood sugar, shouldn't interfere with weight loss, and are also not excitotoxins are stevia, xylitol, and erythritol. Xylitol is extremely toxic to dogs, so if you have a dog, it's best not to keep this in your house. Stevia is part of the ragweed family, and many people with ragweed allergies will find they are allergic to stevia-sweetened products.

Speaking of sweeteners, some of the savory recipes call for a little sweetener to be added. This may seem strange, but in reading labels, you'll find that most spice mixes and sauces have sweetener added. I've found that adding a few drops of monkfruit to some of these recipes adds that something my tastebuds are craving. Of course, you can always omit the sweetener.

Recipes can turn out differently for different people. Our ovens, our ingredients, and our taste buds are all unique. I hope if you try a recipe that doesn't turn out exactly like you expected that you'll try again and make it your own. Also, when cooking with ingredients that are not excitotoxins the change may take a while to get used to.

One last note about the recipes. Due to stringent FDA and USDA guidelines, I have not included nutritional information for the recipes, nor do I make any nutritional claims about any recipe. These are simply recipes I prepared that did not cause me weight gain, but did help me lose weight. There are many apps and websites available to help you calculate nutritional values in foods and recipes, and I encourage you to use such apps and websites to guide you in your weight loss journey.

Hands-off Recipes

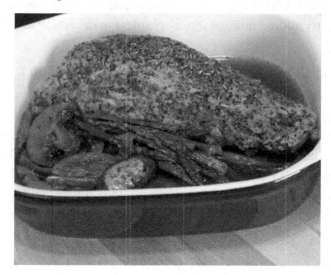

Pork Loin Roast

1 pound pork loin roast

1 tsp. salt

1 tsp. pepper

1 tsp. paprika

1 tsp. thyme

1 tsp. rosemary

1 tsp. garlic powder

1 tsp. onion powder

Make a dry rub by combining salt, pepper, paprika, thyme, rosemary, garlic powder, and onion powder. Rub the spices all over the pork loin. Spray a little olive oil in a skillet and sear the pork loin on each side for 5 minutes per side. Place the pork loin in a baking pan with about a 1/2 inch of broth covering the bottom. Roast at 400°F until internal temperature is 165°F or about 25 minutes.

About this recipe:

Pork loin is a leaner cut of pork. This is a very easy hands-off recipe that goes great with mashed cauliflower, mashed heart of palms, or covered in apple or cranberry sauce. You can even add a jar of sauerkraut to a slow cooker and cook low and slow for an even easier tasty meal.

Cooked pork loin freezes well for about a month. Slice the pork loin into portions and add to freezer bag with one or two wet cotton balls to keep it from drying out. After a month of freezing, it should be served with a topping like applesauce to add moisture.

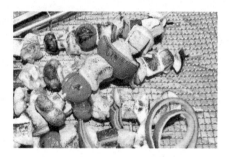

Chicken K-bobs

1-pound cubed chicken

Assorted vegetables cubed

Marinade

1/3 cup Bragg's aminos or low-sodium soy sauce

1/4 cup water

3 Tbsp. lemon juice

2 Tbsp. minced garlic

1 tsp. Italian seasoning

a couple drops of liquid sweetener, or a pinch of no calorie granulated sweetener

Combine all marinade ingredients and let flavors blend. Add cubed chicken to marinade and marinate for at least one hour. While chicken is marinating, wash and cube the vegetables you will be using (squash, zucchini, cherry tomatoes, onion, and mushrooms are good low-fat, low-calorie, nutrient dense options). Preheat oven to 450° and assemble k-bobs. Place in oven on foil lined baking sheet, and turning once, cook until internal temperature of the chicken is 165° (25-30 min.). Broil last ten minutes for a grilled effect.

About this recipe:

The raw, cubed chicken can be frozen for at least a month. This marinade is mild, so while I usually don't recommend freezing chicken in the marinade, I think it works great with this. Freezing in the marinade keeps the chicken from drying out.

The great thing about k-bobs is that you can create one meal but make each k-bob special for every family member. Adding potatoes, is a favorite for my family, and I'll even add some sweet potatoes or radishes to mine on occasion.

Green Chili Pork Stew

<u>Protein</u>

1 lb. pork tenderloin cubed

<u>Sauce</u>

6 tomatillos baked, boiled, or microwaved to soften

14 oz. canned green chilis

1/3 cup jalapeños or 3 Tbsp. green tabasco (optional)

1 Tbsp. garlic powder

1 Tbsp. onion powder

1 Tbsp. lime juice

Place cubed tenderloin in a large pot and brown in broth on medium. Whir all sauce ingredients in blender. Add the sauce to the browned pork and simmer until pork is tender and cooked through.

About this recipe:

This recipe freezes well raw or cooked. To give the pork more flavor, I sometimes marinate it in lime juice, garlic, and onion powder during the day. I've added riced cauliflower to this dish to get more vegetables in, and it was delicious. Once the tomatillo/chili sauce is blended, it's a simple, hands-off recipe that frees you up to work on another dish or spend time with your family. So, make up that sauce ahead of time, freeze it, and thaw it when you're ready for an easy dish!

For the family, this makes delicious green chili pork enchiladas! For enchiladas, bake the pork loin whole, shred the pork, and wrap with tortillas. Cover with the green chili sauce and add any type of cheese your family enjoys. Heat up until the cheese is melted.

Meatloaf

1 pound very lean ground beef, turkey, or pork

1/4 cup egg whites

1/4 cup unsweetened ketchup

1/4 cup mustard

1/2 diced onion sautéed

1/2 medium zucchini shredded

1 Tbsp. Bragg's aminos or low-sodium soy sauce

1 tsp. salt (optional)

1 tsp. pepper

Mix all ingredients together and cook at 350° until internal temperature is 165° (about 1 hour).

About this recipe

This is a tasty but leaner meatloaf version that will satisfy your taste buds and fill you up. The zucchini and onion keep it moist, while the egg whites act as a binder.

The unsweetened ketchup should be a very healthy brand with no sucralose. I prefer Primal Kitchen brand.

This freezes well for a couple of months if needed. It's best to portion out the meatloaf before freezing and start to thaw in the refrigerator one to two days before eating.

I love to eat this with mashed cauliflower or mashed heart of palm. My family enjoys the meatloaf with a side of mashed potatoes or a baked potato. I also like to add a little extra unsweetened ketchup to the top just before serving.

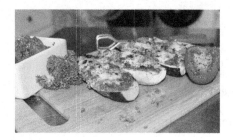

Lasagna Boats

1-pound very lean ground beef, turkey, or pork

4 medium zucchini or yellow squash sliced in half lengthwise and cored out with ends still intact

3/4 cups of your favorite spaghetti sauce (I prefer Rao's)

3/4 cups 1% cottage cheese mixed with 1 tsp. salt, 1 tsp. pepper, and 1 Tbsp. Italian spices

4 teaspoons smoked paprika

3 teaspoons minced garlic

1 teaspoon ground fennel

2 teaspoons pepper

1 tsp. salt (optional)

a small pinch of cayenne pepper and red pepper flakes (optional)

Mix spices together and add ground meat to mix thoroughly. Divide into 8 equal amounts and press into cored out squash halves. Add a little broth to cover the bottom of a baking dish. Top with spaghetti sauce. Cover with foil and bake at 350°F until turkey (or other meat) reaches 165°F. Remove foil when turkey reaches 145°F and add cottage cheese mixture to the tops. Only add cottage cheese when not freezing. Let cottage cheese melt while internal temperature climbs to 165°F. For added vegetables, top with cherry tomatoes and sliced onions cooked with the boats.

About this recipe

This is a leaner version of Italian sausage that will make your taste buds happy! The cottage cheese doesn't freeze very well, so only add cottage cheese when not freezing the boats. This freezes and defrosts well for a few weeks.

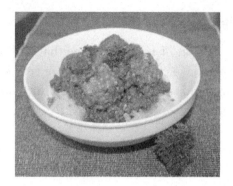

Spaghetti Squash with Meatballs

1-pound very lean ground beef, turkey, or pork

1 small spaghetti squash or frozen spaghetti squash

3 teaspoons smoked paprika

2 teaspoons minced garlic

1 teaspoon ground fennel

2 teaspoons pepper

1 tsp. salt (optional)

Preheat oven to 400°. Rinse spaghetti squash and place on a foil-lined baking dish whole. Cook until it is soft when pushed down and has a large brown spot on the bottom (about an hour and a half). Let cool slightly, slice in half, remove seeds, and pull the squash strands out with a fork.

Combine all spice ingredients in a large bowl and blend completely. Add ground meat to the bowl and mix with hands until the spices are evenly distributed through the ground meat. Form 12 equally sized meatballs and bake in oven until internal temperature reaches 165° (about a half hour). Top with your favorite healthy spaghetti sauce.

About this recipe

These Italian sausage meatballs are delicious as any other meatballs, but they don't have the starches and excitotoxins you'll find in the store bought version, or even other recipes. They will work well for you over your choice of pasta substitute, my favorite is spaghetti squash. Just top with your favorite healthy spaghetti sauce, and you've got a delicious meal! Adding cottage cheese to your sauce is a tasty way to add more protein to this dish. Your family will enjoy these over regular pasta or on hoagie rolls for a meatball sub. The meatballs freeze and thaw very well for weeks.

Baked Chicken Curry

1 pound chicken breasts

1 small red onion chunked

3/4 cups plain, low-fat Greek yogurt

3 Tbsp. tomato paste

1/2 Tbsp. lemon juice

1 tsp. minced garlic

1 tsp. curry powder

1/2 tsp. ginger powder

1/2 tsp. cumin

1/2 tsp. paprika

1/2 tsp. turmeric powder

1/2 tsp. coriander powder

1/4 tsp. cayenne pepper (optional)

2 tsp. salt (optional)

1 small jalapeño seeded

1/2 cup chopped cilantro

Add all ingredients but cilantro to a blender and blend until smooth. Pour this mixture into a gallon storage bag. Cut slits into each chicken breast, add to marinade, and coat completely. Refrigerate for at least 2 hours, preferably overnight.

Preheat the oven to 350°F. Place the chicken pieces side by side (with the marinade) in a baking dish. Cover the pan with aluminum foil and place the baking dish on the center rack of the oven. Bake until internal temperature of chicken reaches 155°, turning chicken halfway through the cooking process (about 1 hour in all).

Remove foil, turn oven broiler on high, and let the chicken broil for a couple minutes. Flip pieces over and broil again for 5 or 6 minutes, or until the chicken is nicely browned.

Use kitchen shears or a pizza slicer to chop up cilantro for garnish.

About this recipe

Enjoy over riced cauliflower or riced hearts of palm.

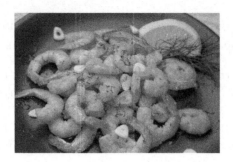

Lemon-Garlic Baked Shrimp

1 pound shrimp deveined and thawed

2 Tbsp. lemon juice

2 Tbsp. sliced or minced garlic

1/2 tsp. onion powder

1/2 tsp. oregano

fresh dill for garnish

1/2 tsp. salt (optional)

Cooking spray

Combine all ingredients in a large bowl and toss shrimp until coated with mixture. Lightly spray a baking sheet with cooking spray. Spread the shrimp around the baking sheet and lightly spray top with cooking spray. Bake at 350° for about five minutes.

About this recipe

This is a nice light recipe that goes well with a shrimp sauce. If your weight loss program tolerates a little fat, you can add butter for a heavier dish with extra flavor.

Shrimp Sauce

1/2 cup unsweetened ketchup (Primal Kitchen is my choice)

2 Tbsp. horseradish

1 Tbsp. lemon juice

1 tsp. hot sauce (Frank's is my choice)

1/2 tsp Bragg's aminos

Mix all ingredients together and enjoy!

Baked Italian Fish

1 pound cod fish filets

8 oz. diced tomato

1 small onion diced and sautéed

4 tsp. minced garlic

1/2 tsp. Italian seasoning

1/4 tsp. salt

1/4 tsp. paprika

2 Tbsp. lemon juice

Broth to cover bottom of baking dish

Minced basil or garlic for garnish

Combine spice ingredients with lemon juice in a zip gallon storage bag. Add fish to bag and coat completely letting marinate for 15-30 minutes. Lightly spray baking dish and pour enough broth in dish to cover bottom of dish. Sauté onions while fish marinates. Add fish, sautéed onion and diced tomatoes to dish and cover with foil. Bake covered at 350 degrees for about 25 minutes.

About this recipe

This is a light, mildly seasoned dish. I enjoy eating this when I need protein, but I'm not very hungry. It goes well with a nice big fresh salad and zucchini or asparagus. Most fish will have been frozen before purchased, and freezing a second time can change the texture. For this reason, I like to prep the marinade ahead of time, and cook the thawed fish when we are ready to eat.

Chocolate Muffins

2 scoops (or 4Tbsp.) of your favorite rice or pea protein powder

1/2 cup egg whites

4 Tbsp. water, almond milk, or other high protein milk replacement

2 Tbsp. cocoa powder

3 Tbsp. granulated sugar substitute

2 tsp. vanilla

2 tsp. baking powder

Add all ingredients to a bowl and blend completely. Add four muffin liners to a muffin tin. Lightly spray muffin liners and divide mixture evenly into liners (12 muffins). Bake at 350° for 25 min.

About this recipe

This can also be made into a mug cake by placing half the recipe into a mug and microwaving for 45-60 seconds. These store well in the refrigerator for days and are great warmed up in the microwave. If you have a strong sweet tooth, you may need to double the amount of sweetener.

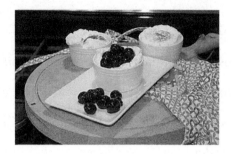

Cottage Cheesecake

1 1/2 cups 1% cottage cheese

3/4 cups nonfat Greek yogurt

1 cup egg whites (or eggs)

1 packet Knox gelatin

1/2 cup monkfruit with erythritol or other granulated sugar replacement

Pour into springform pan or divide into separate ramekins. Bake at 350° for 30-35 minutes. Let cool in refrigerator at 2-4 hours before serving.

About this recipe

This is by far my favorite recipe in the book! I eat this for breakfast a lot. If I really feel like I need a dessert, I'll eat half a serving of cheesecake for dessert. For topping I use frozen organic blueberries or cherries. I simply warm the fruit on the stove or in the microwave, add a little monk fruit sweetener then pour over the top. I enjoy this crustless, but if you really feel you need a crust, you can make a nutrient packed, high protein crust using your favorite pea protein powder.

Protein Powder Cheesecake Crust

1 cup pea protein powder

1/3 cup monkfruit with erythritol or other granulated sugar replacement

1/2 cup egg whites

1/4-1/3 cup water

Combine protein powder with sugar replacement then add egg whites. Start adding water a little at a time until you get a clay consistency that holds together well. Press into the bottom of a dish or springform pan that has been coated with cooking spray. Pour cheesecake mixture on top and cook according to cheesecake recipe.

About this recipe

This crust will not have the texture of a traditional cheesecake crust, but it is a healthy alternative. Choose a protein powder with a taste you love, and this will satisfy your taste buds!

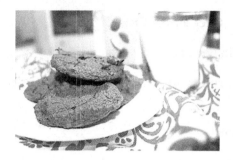

Pumpkin Spice Breakfast Cookies

9 oz. canned pumpkin

1 1/4 cups organic rice or pea protein powder

3/4 cups egg whites

4 tsp. pumpkin pie spice

Sweetener to taste (about a 1/2 cup erythritol, 2 tsp. monkfruit liquid, 1 tsp. stevia)

Preheat oven to 400°

Mix all ingredients together. Drop onto a sprayed or parchment paper lined cookie sheet

(16 cookies). Bake for 12-15 minutes or until the edges are slightly golden.

About this recipe

These are a very good replacement for granola bars or other high-fat, high sugar breakfast bars. They are a soft cookie that is a filling treat, and they are perfect to eat on the go. They freeze well and should be placed in the refrigerator to thaw.

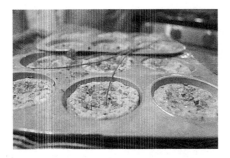

Omelet Muffins

2 cups egg whites

2/3 cup 1% cottage cheese

1/2 cup of your favorite salsa

Combine all ingredients and pour into sprayed muffin tins. Bake at 350° until firm in the center (about 25 minutes).

About this recipe

These muffins turn out like a mini omelet. I like to top mine with sautéed mushrooms and onions to fill me up. They are also delicious topped with extra salsa, and for added protein you can top with nonfat plain Greek yogurt. They freeze well and hold together firm, but some of the moisture will seep out when they thaw.

Hands-on Recipes

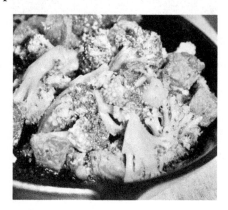

Beef with Broccoli Stir Fry

1 lb. sirloin cubed

16 oz. frozen broccoli florets

1 yellow or white onion diced

Marinade

1/3 cup Bragg's aminos or low sodium soy sauce

2 Tbsp. granulated sugar alternative

1 tsp. ground ginger

1/2 tsp. garlic powder

Combine all marinade ingredients and set aside for flavors to blend. Sauté onions and cubed sirloin on medium until meat is cooked through. While meat is sautéing, heat up frozen broccoli florets in microwave. Once meat has finished cooking, add the marinade to the pan along with the cooked broccoli florets. Toss until all broccoli and beef is coated.

About this recipe

This is a delicious Asian inspired dish. It tastes delicious over riced heart of palm with a little Bragg's or low sodium soy sauce added. To prepare ahead of time, keep the steak and marinade separate, then marinate for 3 hours up to overnight. I usually let this thaw the day before and marinate in the refrigerator throughout the day, then cook up for dinner that evening.

Barbecue Chicken

1 pound chicken breasts

1/2 cup unsweetened ketchup (Primal kitchen is the brand I prefer)

3 Tbsp. granulated sugar substitute

1 Tbsp. apple cider vinegar

1/2 Tbsp. Bragg's Aminos or low-sodium soy sauce

1/2 Tbsp. liquid smoke (look for one with no excitotoxins)

1/2 tsp. garlic powder

1/2 tsp. salt

This recipe is great on the grill, but also turns out well prepared on the stovetop. Pour about 1/4 of an inch of broth in bottom of skillet and heat on medium. Place chicken breasts in skillet and cook covered for five minutes on each side. Cook until internal temperature reaches 165°.

While chicken is cooking, blend barbecue sauce ingredients. Once chicken is browned on both sides and cooked through completely, pour barbecue sauce over the chicken and heat.

About this recipe

Cooking the chicken in a pan lends itself to a very tender chicken breast. When freezing, you will want to freeze the chicken with the barbecue sauce to retain the moisture. The chicken can easily be shredded for barbecue chicken sandwiches by placing in a stand mixer and adding more barbecue sauce as needed.

Sweet and Sour Chicken

1 lb. cubed chicken breast

<u>Marinade</u>

4 tsp. minced garlic

1/2 cup unsweetened ketchup

1/2 cup water

2 tsp. liquid monkfruit sweetener or ¼ cup erythritol

2 Tbsp. apple cider vinegar

2 tsp. Bragg's aminos

1/2 tsp. sea salt

1/2 tsp pepper

Add marinade ingredients to gallon storage bag. Cube chicken and add to marinade. Marinate for at least one hour. Scoop chicken into frying pan from the storage bag while leaving as much marinade as possible in the bag. Cook over medium heat until chicken is cooked to 165°, adding chicken broth or water as needed. When chicken is cooked through, add remaining marinade to coat the chicken and cook until the temperature also reaches 165°.

About this recipe:

The marinade freezes very well, so you can make it ahead of time. Cube the chicken and store raw, separate from the marinade. Move both the chicken and the marinade to the refrigerator to start thawing a day or two before you are ready to cook the meal. Marinate the chicken for at least an hour, but overnight will taste even better. I like this best with riced heart of palm, but for food rotation and cost savings, I often eat it riced cauliflower and add a little Bragg's aminos to the cauliflower for more flavor.

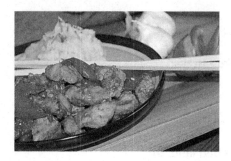

Sweet Chili Pork

1 pound pork loin cubed

2 diced red bell peppers

Marinade

4 Tbsp. chili garlic sauce (reduce for a milder dish)

6 Tbsp. white rice vinegar

1 tsp. paprika

2 tsp. onion powder

30 drops or 1/4 cup granulated sugar replacement

1/2 cup water

Blend all marinade ingredients together and place half in a gallon storage bag. Place the cubed pork loin and bell pepper into the bag to marinate for at least one hour. When done marinating, cook in frying pan on medium heat until meat is cooked through, and peppers are tender. Add the remaining half of marinade to pan and coat meat completely.

About this recipe:

Be sure to marinate the pepper with the meat for at least one hour. I've frozen the uncooked meat in the marinade with the peppers and let it thaw for 24 hours before cooking it all in the frying pan when I got home from work. It was amazing! It turns out sweet and spicy. White rice vinegar gives it a more mellow and sweet taste than regular white vinegar, but regular vinegar will work in a pinch.

If you or family don't like spicy foods, reduce the amount of red garlic chili sauce by at least half. I don't consider this to be spicy, but my husband does. Everyone has different taste buds, so you may need to experiment. I like to eat this with riced heart of palm and a nice refreshing side salad.

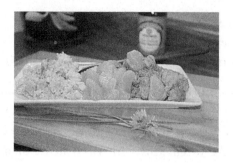

Orange-Ginger Chicken

1 pound chicken breast cut into small pieces

12 ounces of mandarin oranges

2 thumbs of fresh ginger

1/4 cup Bragg's aminos (add broth or water to thin)

Cut up chicken and place in frying pan with broth. Cook over medium heat until chicken is cooked to 165°, adding chicken broth or water as needed. When chicken is cooked through, add ginger, Bragg's aminos and oranges. Stir to coat chicken and heat oranges.

About this recipe:

The Bragg's aminos are strong flavored, so don't marinate the chicken. This hands-on recipe requires some attention to be sure the chicken isn't overcooked, and the oranges don't become mushy. I like to eat this over riced cauliflower or riced hearts of palm, while my family eats this over white rice. To prepare ahead of time, keep the marinade separate from the chicken. Oranges can be frozen for about a week without changing the texture.

Salsa Steak

1 pound sirloin cut into large pieces

16 oz. jar of your favorite healthy salsa

10 oz. can diced tomatoes and green chilis

2 Tbsp. minced garlic

2 Tbsp. lime juice

1/2 Tbsp. Bragg's aminos or low sodium soy sauce

Broth to thin while cooking

Cover the bottom of a frying pan with broth and cook cubed sirloin until browned. Add garlic and sauté for one minute to bring out the flavor. Add all remaining ingredients and heat through. If all ingredients were frozen together, cook everything together and add broth as needed to cook until sirloin is cooked through.

About this recipe

This all freezes well together and can be cooked together for a great time saver. The tomato and chili won't overpower the steak, so the steak can stay in the marinade for days. Salsa steak is delicious served with riced cauliflower or healthy tortillas.

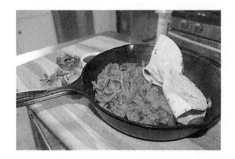

Fajitas

1 pound sirloin, chicken, or pork loin tenderized and cut into strips

2 red, yellow, orange, or green bell peppers sliced

1 sliced onion

1 tsp. salt

1 tsp. paprika

1 tsp. onion powder

1 tsp. garlic powder

1 tsp. cumin

1 tsp. coriander

1/4-1/2 tsp. cayenne pepper

a few drops of liquid sweetener

Combine all ingredients in a plastic gallon storage bag, then set bag aside for flavors to blend. Place meat, onions, and peppers into marinade and let marinate for at least one hour. Sauté all ingredients on medium in large pan until onions and peppers are tender and meat is cooked through.

About this recipe

This recipe makes a mild fajita meat that is good served in healthy tortillas or over salad. To prepare ahead of time, you can freeze the sirloin or pork, onions, and peppers with the marinade. If using chicken, freeze the marinade separate, then marinate chicken for at least one hour before cooking.

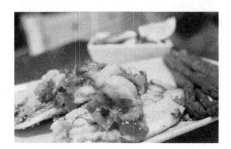

Mango Salsa Tilapia

1 pound tilapia filets

3 tsp. chili powder

2 tsp. garlic powder

1/2 tsp. salt

2 Tbsp. lime juice

1 tsp. lime zest

Cooking broth

Combine marinade ingredients in a plastic gallon storage bag. Place the fish in the bag and let marinate for 15-30 minutes. Use non-stick pan to fry in broth or lightly oiled pan. Cook about 4 minutes on each side until fish is flaky.

About this recipe

Most fish will have been frozen before it gets to our stores and freezing a second time can change the texture. For this reason, I like to prepare the marinade and salsa ahead of time and thaw the frozen fish the day it will be eaten. If your family likes fish tacos, this recipe is perfect! You will enjoy it without the tortillas if that's what your weight loss plan requires, and your family will enjoy this with tortillas and other toppings. Mixing your favorite hot sauce with Greek yogurt is also delicious side to eat with this recipe.

Mango Salsa – makes enough salsa for 1 pound of fish

1 cup cubed mango

3 Tbsp. red bell peppers

3 Tbsp. chopped cilantro

1 tsp. jalapeños

1 1/2 Tbsp. lime juice

Combine all ingredients and let set for about an hour.

About this recipe

Mango salsa will last in the refrigerator for up to 3 days in a glass container, so you can easily rotate foods by saving some salsa to eat later in the week.

Chili

1-pound very lean ground beef, turkey, or pork

1 cup white onion, diced

1 cup stewed tomatoes

1 diced red bell pepper

1 jar sliced mushrooms

6 Tbsp. chili powder (more if needed)

2 Tbsp. onion powder

2 Tbsp. garlic powder

1 Tbsp. salt (optional)

Broth for browning meat

Brown meat in saucepan with broth, salt, onion powder, and garlic powder. Add all remaining ingredients, simmer until flavors blend together.

About this recipe

This is a very filling comfort food for me and my family. When we eat chili, I will usually make cornbread for the family, and I will toast some low-calorie bread for myself. The chili freezes very well for weeks, and turns out great thawed in the microwave or refrigerator.

Lemon-Garlic Fish

1 cup minced fresh parsley

2/3 cup lemon juice

3 Tbsp. minced garlic

½ tsp. salt

½ tsp. pepper

Combine marinade ingredients in a plastic gallon storage bag. Place the fish in the bag and let marinate for 15-30 minutes. Use non-stick pan to fry in broth or lightly oiled pan. Cook about 4 minutes on each side until fish is flaky.

About this recipe

Most fish will have been frozen before it gets to our stores and freezing a second time can change the texture. For this reason, I like to prepare the marinade ahead of time and thaw the frozen fish the day it will be eaten. I like this dish with asparagus and fresh fruit.

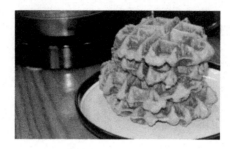

Protein Waffles

makes 4 waffles

1/2 cup canned pumpkin

1/4-1/2 cup pea protein powder

1/4 cup egg whites

1 tsp. baking powder

1/2 tsp. monkfruit drops or 1 Tbsp. granulated sugar replacement (Lakanto is my choice)

1/2 tsp. vanilla

Mix all ingredients together to make a thick batter. Add more protein powder to thicken the batter if needed. Be sure to spray waffle iron with cooking spray for every waffle, otherwise they will stick. Spread the mixture onto the middle of the waffle iron. Cook according to waffle iron instructions. Top with warmed fruit you have added sugar alternative to instead of using syrup.

About this recipe

Protein waffles can be made with a variety ingredients including Greek yogurt and rice protein powder. My favorite recipe is the pumpkin and pea protein version. I think the texture and flavor are better, but try adding different things to see which you prefer.

These are a more delicate waffle than traditional waffles and will fall apart easily if the waffle maker is not sprayed every time. They freeze very well, and can easily be heated up in the toaster. If you must have syrup with your waffles, try to find a low calorie syrup without sucralose or maltodextrin as both have been shown to interfere with blood sugar levels which can make you more hungry. Lakanto makes a great, syrup replacement. I usually top my waffles with fruit that has been cooked with sweetener.

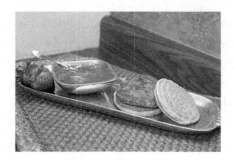

MockGriddles

MockGriddle Muffins – makes 6 muffins

6 Tbsp. of your favorite pea protein powder

6 ounces of egg white

3 tsp. maple extract

2 tsp. baking powder

1/4 cup erythritol or 20 drops liquid sweetener

Combine all ingredients to create a thick batter. Preheat frying pan on medium. Spray large mason jar lid rings with cooking spray. Pour 1/4 cup of mix into each lid to make six muffins. Flip when muffins bubble at the top. Once flipped, use a fork to remove the lid.

About this recipe

Use these with the breakfast sausage recipe to make your own version of the popular fast food breakfast! These freeze very well, heat up well in the microwave or toaster, and are a great breakfast when you're on the go.

Breakfast Sausage - 3 servings

1-pound lean ground pork

3 tsp. paprika

3 tsp. garlic (minced or crushed)

2 tsp. pepper

1 1/2 tsp. salt

1 tsp. ground fennel

Mix the spices together in a bowl and add the ground pork to the spices and combine. Heat up broth in a non-stick frying pan and fry up ground, or cook into patties for 2-3 minutes on each side until browned and cooked through.

Protein Pancakes

makes 1 large or 2 small pancakes

1/4 cup organic pea protein powder

2 ounces egg whites

1 tsp. baking powder

Water to thin

Cook protein mixture in a non-stick skillet that has been sprayed with cooking spray, flipping once bubbles start to form on the tops of the pancakes. Cook until golden brown, about 30-60 seconds. Top pancake with cooked, sweetened berries instead of syrup.

About this recipe

In place of syrup, I like to heat up frozen berries in the microwave, add a little monkfruit, and pour over the pancakes. If you must have syrup with your pancakes, try to find a low calorie syrup without sucralose or maltodextrin as both have been shown to interfere with blood sugar levels which can make you more hungry. Lakanto makes a great syrup replacement.

12

TEMPERATURES, WEIGHTS, AND NUMBERS

There are a number of gadgets that are really important for meal planning. They make our lives easy, and they make the whole meal-prepping process less daunting. The biggest of these, such as slow cookers, freezers, and refrigerators, have temperature requirements that we need to adhere too. This chapter will help you navigate the cooking and freezing temperatures for various foods.

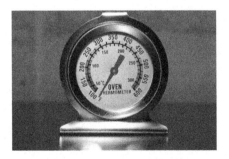

Slow Cooker

A broad variety of slow cookers are available. It's important to read the instruction booklet that came with yours, so you are clear on its specifications. Temperatures and time frames for setup may differ depending on the manufacturer. So, to be considered a safe slow cooker, your gadget must be able to cook food slowly enough for it to be left unattended and fast enough to keep food hot enough for it to be above the danger zone.

When using a slow cooker, keep the following in mind:

- Begin with fresh or thawed meat rather than frozen.
- Instead of huge chops or roasts, use pieces. Use poultry chunks rather than a whole chicken.
- Cook the meat on high for an hour, then reduce to low, rather than cooking on low for the entire time.
- Use only recipes that incorporate a liquid. For optimal results, fill the cooker to 12%–34% of its capacity.
- Check the interior temperature of the meal to ensure it reaches 160 °F.
- Do not postpone the alter the cooking time of the recipe.
- Do not reheat food in a slow cooker.
- Preheat the slow cooker for about 20 minutes before adding food.
- Keep the lid closed.

The following table shows the food loads and cooking times for typical slow cookers:

Cut	Weight	Cook Time (Low Temp)	Cook Time (High Temp)
Poultry	6 pounds	7 1/2 hours	6 1/4 hours
Beef roast	3–4 pounds	8 hours	5 3/4 hours
Fish	2 pounds	3 1/2 hours	1 1/2 hours
Pork loin	3–4 pounds	6 hours	5 hours
Pork roast (large)	6–7 pounds	9 1/2 hours	7 1/3 hours
Meat stew	3 pounds	6 hours	4 3/4 hours

These cooking times are estimated and vary depending on individual meat features, such as fat content and connective tissue, as well as other components of the meal, such as meat cube size, amount of liquid, the way the slow cooker is packed, and so on.

Temperatures and Roasting Times

To ensure that meat and poultry have achieved an acceptable minimum internal temperature, always use a food thermometer. Set the oven temperature to 325 °F or higher when roasting meat and poultry. Always cook raw poultry and meat to an accepted internal minimum temperature.

Below are the optimal roasting temperatures for beef and pork:

Roast	Weight	Oven Temperature	Internal Minimum Temperature When Cooked	Total Cooking Time
Round tip roast (sirloin)	3–4 pounds	325 °F	140 °F	Medium rare: 1 3/4–2 hours
			155 °F	Medium: 2 1/4–2 1/2 hours
	4–6 pounds		140 °F	Medium rare: 2–2 1/2 hours
			155 °F	Medium: 2 1/2–3 hours
Pork tenderloin roast	2–3 pounds	425 °F	135 °F	Medium rare: 35–40 minutes
			150 °F	Medium: 45–50 minutes
	4–5 pounds		135 °F	Medium rare: 50–60 minutes
			150 °F	Medium: 60–70 minutes

And the following are the optimal poultry roasting temperatures:

Bird	Weight	Oven Temperature	Cooking Times
Chicken, broiler/fryer (defrosted and without stuffing)	3–4 pounds	350 °F	1 1/4–1 1/2 hours
	5–7 pounds	350 °F	2–2 1/4 hours
Whole turkey (defrosted and without stuffing	8–12 pounds	325 °F	2 3/4–3 hours
	12–14 pounds	325 °F	3–3 3/4 hours
	14–18 pounds	325 °F	3 3/4–4 1/4 hours
	18–20 pounds	325 °F	4 1/4–4 1/2 hours

Refrigerator and Freezer

Freezing doesn't improve the flavor or texture of any food, but it can preserve the majority of the fresh product's quality when done at the right temperature and for the right duration. To retain quality, food should be frozen at 0 °F. These guidelines will assist in preventing refrigerated food at 40 °F from spoiling or becoming dangerous.

Here are some important tips when buying meat and poultry:

- Buy the item before the expiration date.
- Follow the product's handling instructions.
- Keep meat and poultry in their original packaging until just before use.
- If freezing meat or poultry in its original package for more than 2 months, wrap it in airtight heavy-duty foil, plastic wrap, or freezer paper, or place it inside a plastic bag.

Figuring out the length of time a food item can be kept in the refrigerator or freezer before it goes bad is not always straightforward.

The following table shows guidelines for refrigerator and freezer temperatures:

Food	Type	Refrigerator	Freezer
Fresh veal, beef, pork, lamb	Uncooked	3–5 days	4–12 months
	Cooked	3–4 days	2–6 months
	Ground	1–2 days	3–4 months
Fresh poultry	Whole raw chicken or turkey	1–2 days	1 year
	Raw chicken or turkey pieces	1–2 days	9 months
	Cooked	3–4 days	2–6 months
	Ground	1–2 days	3–4 months
Fish	Fatty fish (tuna, salmon, catfish, mackerel)	1–3 days	2–3 months
	Lean fish (halibut, cod, sole)		6–8 months
	Other fish (sea trout, pollock, rockfish)		4–8 months
Eggs	Raw eggs	3–5 weeks	To freeze, beat the egg first
	Uncooked yolks and egg whites	2–4 days	Yolks do not freeze well. Egg whites can be frozen for 12 months
	Hard-boiled eggs	1 week	Should not be frozen
	Quiche, baked	3–5 days	2–3 months
Stews and soups	With vegetables and/or meat	3–4 days	2–3 months

In Chapter 2 we talked about some of the benefits of low-glycemic foods—you stay full longer, and they curb cravings. Remember, low glycemic index foods are rated a 55 or below and low glycemic load foods are rated a 10 or below. The lower the number, the better, and when both numbers are low, you've found a food that can help with weight loss.

Low glycemic foods take longer to digest, leading to balanced blood sugar levels; high glycemic foods digest fast and cause a rapid increase in blood sugar levels. Here is the glycemic index of common foods to help you determine if the food you're eating is a low-, medium-, or high-glycemic food:

Type of Food	Glycemic Index	Glycemic Load
Pear	38	4
Grapefruit	25	3
Orange	42	5
Banana	62	16
Apples	39	6
Peach	42	5
Mango	51	5
Pineapple	59	8
Pumpkin	64	7
Carrots	16	1
Green Peas	51	4
Russet Potato	111	33
Sweet Potato	70	20
Cupcake	73	19
Pancakes	66	17
White Rice	64	28
Brown Rice	66	21
Bagel	69	24
Pretzels	83	16

13

CONCLUSION

L osing weight is not easy, and staying on course can be a challenge, but with a bit of planning it can be achieved. As mentioned a few times throughout the book, there's no right or wrong way of planning and prepping. Find a plan that works for you, your family, and your lifestyle. The plans in this book are not cast in stone; they are a foundation from which you can create a plan that is uniquely you.

In this book we covered four meal-prep plans:

- The once-and-done meal-prep plan, which allows you to plan and prep meals for the entire week in 3 or fewer hours
- The power-hour meal-prep plan, for people who can spare only an hour for meal-prep planning
- The batch-cooking meal-prep plan, for people who want to plan and prep enough meals for the entire month
- The hybrid meal-prep plan, which allows you to mix and match the three plans to create your own

It is important to remember that for successful and stress-free meal prepping, you need to be organized. Make sure all the equipment you are going to use is within reach; trying to find where things are at the last minute (and with greasy hands) will frustrate you and mess with your momentum. Create a mini assembly line before you start; this way you will quickly spot if a tool, spice, or piece of equipment is missing.

When it comes to choosing your ingredients, keep in mind that the quality of your ingredients has an impact on the final product and also affects how long you can keep the food in the fridge or freezer.

Even though the primary goal of your meal prep is weight loss, design your meals in such a manner that the nutritional needs of all members of your household are met. For instance, if you have children, you could include some additional protein-rich foods for their development phases. Also, you can prepare the same meal to meet the needs of both overweight and underweight family members by adding and removing certain elements.

In this book you'll find tools to help you on your journey. These include meat-cooking temperature charts, freezer and refrigerator temperature charts, and a food glycemic chart to help you take the guesswork out of meal prepping.

The information in this book is meant to help you create and design meal-prep plans that are appropriate for you and your family. Use it as a foundation and for encouragement on those days when you lack the inspiration to meal prep.

GLOSSARY

Electrolytes: Chemicals that, when dissolved in water, conduct electricity. Electrolytes are required for a variety of bodily activities.

Excitotoxins: A class of chemicals that overstimulate neuron receptors, stimulating taste cells and making food seem irresistable.

FDA: The food and drug administration in the United States, responsible for protecting the public health.

Glucose-dependent insulinotropic peptide: A hormone that increases insulin secretion after eating. It is produced by the small intestine.

Glucose-like peptide 1: A hormone secreted by the intestines in reaction to eating. It reduces appetite and causes insulin to be released.

Glycemic Index: A number given to foods, used to assess the relative insulin response burden of a food.

Glycemic Load: A number given to foods that uses the amount of carbohydrate in a food to determine how quickly the food will raise blood glucose levels.

USDA: The United States Department of Agriculture, responsible for regulating and protecting U.S. agricultural health.

REFERENCES

Assistant Secretary for Public Affairs (ASPA. (2019, June 24). *Cold food storage chart*. FoodSafety.gov. https://www.foodsafety.gov/food-safety-charts/cold-food-storage-charts

Baik I, Lee M, Jun NR, Lee JY, Shin C. A healthy dietary pattern consisting of a variety of food choices is inversely associated with the development of metabolic syndrome. Nutr Res Pract. 2013 Jun;7(3):233-41. doi: 10.4162/nrp.2013.7.3.233. Epub 2013 Jun 3. PMID: 23766885; PMCID: PMC3679333.

Barnett, B. (n.d.). *Do men lose weight faster than women?* WebMD. https://www.webmd.com/diet/features/do-men-lose-weight-faster-than-women

Bentley-Lewis, R., Koruda, K., & Seely, E. W. (2007). The metabolic syndrome in women. *Nature Clinical Practice. Endocrinology & Metabolism, 3*(10), 696–704. https://doi.org/10.1038/ncpendmet0616

Bertoia, M. L., Mukamal, K. J., Cahill, L. E., Hou, T., Ludwig, D. S., Mozaffarian, D., Willett, W. C., Hu, F. B., & Rimm, E. B. (2015). Changes in intake of fruits and vegetables and weight change in

United States men and women followed for up to 24 years: Analysis from three prospective cohort studies. *PLOS Medicine, 12*(9), e1001878. https://doi.org/10.1371/journal.pmed.1001878

Bethene, E. R. (2009). *Prevalence of metabolic syndrome among adults 20 years of age and over, by sex, age, race and ethnicity, and body mass index; United States, 2003–2006.* Centers for Disease Control and Prevention. https://stacks.cdc.gov/view/cdc/5448

Campbell, C., & Olsen, C. O. (2020, January 14). *The 10 best tools to help you meal prep successfully.* Reviewed. https://www.reviewed.com/cooking/features/the-10-best-tools-to-meal-prep-successfully

Christensen, P., Meinert Larsen, T., Westerterp-Plantenga, M., Macdonald, I., Martinez, J. A., Handjiev, S., Poppitt, S., Hansen, S., Ritz, C., Astrup, A., Pastor-Sanz, L., Sandø-Pedersen, F., Pietiläinen, K. H., Sundvall, J., Drummen, M., Taylor, M. A., Navas-Carretero, S., Handjieva-Darlenska, T., Brodie, S., & Silvestre, M. P. (2018). Men and women respond differently to rapid weight loss: Metabolic outcomes of a multi-centre intervention study after a low-energy diet in 2500 overweight individuals with pre-diabetes (PREVIEW). *Diabetes, Obesity and Metabolism, 20*(12), 2840–2851. https://doi.org/10.1111/dom.13466

Cooking Light. (2018, September 6). *Here's how to properly freeze foods.* Cooking Light. https://www.cookinglight.com/cooking-101/techniques/how-to-freeze-foods?slide=139942#139942

Damsbo-Svendsen, S., Rønsholdt, M. D., & Lauritzen, L. (2013). Fish oil-supplementation increases appetite in healthy adults. A randomized controlled cross-over trial. *Appetite, 66,* 62–66. https://doi.org/10.1016/j.appet.2013.02.019

David Shadinger, John Katsion, Sue Myllykangas & Denise Case (2020) The Impact of a Positive, Self-Talk Statement on Public Speaking Anxiety, College Teaching, 68:1, 5-11, DOI: 10.1080/87567555.2019.1680522

Du, S., Zhang, H., Wu, H., Ye, S., Li, W., & Su, Q. (2020). Prevalence and gender differences of metabolic syndrome in young ketosis-prone type 2 diabetic individuals: A retrospective Study. *Diabetes, Metabolic Syndrome and Obesity: Targets and Therapy, 13*, 2719–2727. https://doi.org/10.2147/dmso.s252492

Felman, A. (2017, November 20). *Electrolytes: Uses, imbalance, and supplementation.* Www.medicalnewstoday.com. https://www.medical-newstoday.com/articles/153188

Ferrari, N. (2015, February 17). *Making one change—getting more fiber—can help with weight loss.* Harvard Health Blog. https://www.health.harvard.edu/blog/making-one-change-getting-fiber-can-help-weight-loss-201502177721

Fiona S. Atkinson, Kaye Foster-Powell, Jennie C. Brand-Miller; International Tables of Glycemic Index and Glycemic Load Values: 2008. *Diabetes Care* 1 December 2008; 31 (12): 2281–2283. https://doi.org/10.2337/dc08-1239

Food Insight. (2019, July 19). *Everything you need to know about aspartame.* IFIC Foundation. https://foodinsight.org/everything-you-need-to-know-about-aspartame/

Goldman, R. (2016, July 29). *Magnesium for weight loss: Does it help?* Healthline. https://www.healthline.com/health/food-nutrition/magnesium-for-weight-loss

Gunnars, K. (2018). *Protein intake—How much protein should you eat per day?* Healthline. https://www.healthline.com/nutrition/how-much-protein-per-day

Gray, B., Steyn, F., Davies, P. S., & Vitetta, L. (2013). Omega-3 fatty acids: A review of the effects on adiponectin and leptin and potential implications for obesity management. *European Journal of Clinical Nutrition, 67*(12), 1234–1242. https://doi.org/10.1038/ejcn.2013.197

Harvard Health Publishing. (2019). *A good guide to good carbs: The glycemic index—Harvard Health.* Harvard Health; Harvard Health.

https://www.health.harvard.edu/healthbeat/a-good-guide-to-good-carbs-the-glycemic-index

He, K., Du, S., Xun, P., Sharma, S., Wang, H., Zhai, F., & Popkin, B. (2011). Consumption of monosodium glutamate in relation to incidence of overweight in Chinese adults: China health and nutrition survey (CHNS). *The American Journal of Clinical Nutrition, 93*(6), 1328–1336. https://doi.org/10.3945/ajcn.110.008870

John Hopkins Medicine. (2021). *Intermittent fasting: What is it, and how does it work?* Www.hopkinsmedicine.org. https://www.hopkinsmedicine.org/health/wellness-and-prevention/intermittent-fasting-what-is-it-and-how-does-it-work

Johnston, C. S. (2005). Strategies for healthy weight loss: From vitamin C to the glycemic response. *Journal of the American College of Nutrition, 24*(3), 158–165. https://doi.org/10.1080/07315724.2005.10719460

Kaiser Permanente (2008). Keeping A Food Diary Doubles Diet Weight Loss, Study Suggests *ScienceDaily. ScienceDaily, 8 July 2008.* https://www.sciencedaily.com/releases/2008/07/080708080738.htm

Katterman SN, Kleinman BM, Hood MM, Nackers LM, Corsica JA. Mindfulness meditation as an intervention for binge eating, emotional eating, and weight loss: a systematic review. Eat Behav. 2014 Apr;15(2):197-204. doi: 10.1016/j.eatbeh.2014.01.005. Epub 2014 Feb 1. PMID: 24854804.

Leidy HJ, Clifton PM, Astrup A, Wycherley TP, Westerterp-Plantenga MS, Luscombe-Marsh ND, Woods SC, Mattes RD. The role of protein in weight loss and maintenance. Am J Clin Nutr. 2015 Jun;101(6):1320S-1329S. doi: 10.3945/ajcn.114.084038. Epub 2015 Apr 29. PMID: 25926512.

Lennerz, B., & Lennerz, J. K. (2018). Food addiction, high-glycemic-index carbohydrates, and obesity. *Clinical Chemistry, 64*(1), 64–71. https://doi.org/10.1373/clinchem.2017.273532

Li, C., Xing, C., Zhang, J., Zhao, H., Shi, W., & He, B. (2021). Eight-hour time-restricted feeding improves endocrine and metabolic profiles in women with anovulatory polycystic ovary syndrome. *Journal of Translational Medicine, 19.* https://doi.org/10.1186/s12967-021-02817-2

Loucks, E. B., Rehkopf, D. H., Thurston, R. C., & Kawachi, I. (2007). Socioeconomic disparities in metabolic syndrome differ by gender: Evidence from NHANES III. *Annals of Epidemiology, 17*(1), 19–26. https://doi.org/10.1016/j.annepidem.2006.07.002

Malchar Chiropractic & Wellness Center. (2018, October 9). *Baffled by glycemic index vs load?* Malchar Chiropractic & Wellness Center. https://www.malcharwellness.com/blog/2018/10/9/baffled-by-glycemic-index-vs-load

Manzella, D. (2021, October 9). *How the glycemic index chart can help manage blood sugar.* Verywell Health. https://www.verywellhealth.com/glycemic-index-chart-for-common-foods-1087476

Marcus, A. (2011, May 27). MSG linked to weight gain. *Reuters.* https://www.reuters.com/article/us-msg-linked-weight-gain-idUS-TRE74Q5SJ20110527

Marengo, C. (2022, February 11). *Weight loss meal plans: Tips, 7-day menu, and more.* Www.medicalnewstoday.com. https://www.medicalnewstoday.com/articles/weight-loss-meal-plan

MedlinePlus. (2020, January 17). *Metabolic syndrome.* Medlineplus.gov. https://medlineplus.gov/metabolicsyndrome.html

Metabolic Meals. (2016, August 10). *Food rotation for faster fat loss.* Metabolic Meals— Blog. https://blog.mymetabolicmeals.com/food-rotation-for-faster-fat-loss/

Muth, N. (2012, March 21). *Do men and women have different nutritional needs?* Www.acefitness.org. https://www.acefitness.org/resources/everyone/blog/2461/do-men-and-women-have-different-nutritional-needs/

Nast, C. (2016, January 21). *The right way to freeze basically everything.* Bon Appétit. http://www.bonappetit.com/test-kitchen/how-to/article/how-to-freeze-vegetables-soup-meat-fruit

Organic Facts. (2008, March 26). *15 impressive benefits of fennel*. Organic Facts. https://www.organicfacts.net/health-benefits/herbs-and-spices/health-benefits-of-fennel

Otten, J., Ryberg, M., Mellberg, C., Andersson, T., Chorell, E., Lindahl, B., Larsson, C., Holst, J. J., & Olsson, T. (2019). Postprandial levels of GLP-1, GIP and glucagon after 2 years of weight loss with a Paleolithic diet: a randomised controlled trial in healthy obese women. *European Journal of Endocrinology*, *180*(6), 417–427. https://doi.org/10.1530/EJE-19-0082

Parra, D., Ramel, A., Bandarra, N., Kiely, M., Martínez, J. A., & Thorsdottir, I. (2008). A diet rich in long chain omega-3 fatty acids modulates satiety in overweight and obese volunteers during weight loss. *Appetite, 51*(3), 676–680. https://doi.org/10.1016/j.appet.2008.06.003

Petre, A. (2017, September 12). *Can omega-3 fish oil help you lose weight?* Healthline. https://www.healthline.com/nutrition/omega-3-fish-oil-and-weight-loss

Rama, M., & Miller, B. (2016, March 26). *Roasting times and temperatures for poultry and meat*. Dummies. https://www.dummies.com/article/home-auto-hobbies/food-drink/cooking-baking/general-cooking-baking/roasting-times-and-temperatures-for-poultry-and-meat-146873/

Raman, R. (2017, April 2). *How eating fiber can help you lose belly fat*. Healthline; Healthline Media. https://www.healthline.com/nutrition/fiber-and-belly-fat

Sadri Damirchi E, Mojarrad A, Pireinaladin S, Grjibovski AM. The Role of Self-Talk in Predicting Death Anxiety, Obsessive-Compulsive Disorder, and Coping Strategies in the Face of Coronavirus Disease (COVID-19). Iran J Psychiatry. 2020 Jul;15(3):182-188. doi: 10.18502/ijp-s.v15i3.3810. PMID: 33193766; PMCID: PMC7603592.

Seaver, V. (2020, June 12). *The essential meal-prep tools you need in your kitchen, according to a meal-prep pro.* EatingWell. https://www.eatingwell.com/article/7825137/the-essential-tools-you-need-in-your-kitchen-for-meal-prep/

Slavin JL, Lloyd B. Health benefits of fruits and vegetables. Adv Nutr. 2012 Jul 1;3(4):506-16. doi: 10.3945/an.112.002154. PMID: 22797986; PMCID: PMC3649719.

St John, A. (2020, August 14). *How much protein do your athletes really need?* Science for Sport. https://www.scienceforsport.com/how-much-protein-do-your-athletes-really-need/

Tarantino, O. (2016, September 18). *34 tips for freezing food.* Eat This Not That. https://www.eatthis.com/tips-for-freezing-food/

Thom G, Lean MEJ, Brosnahan N, Algindan YY, Malkova D, Dombrowski SU. 'I have been all in, I have been all out and I have been everything in-between': A 2-year longitudinal qualitative study of weight loss maintenance. J Hum Nutr Diet. 2021 Feb;34(1):199-214. doi: 10.1111/jhn.12826. Epub 2020 Oct 21. PMID: 33089558.

U.S. Department of Agriculture, Agricultural Research Service. FoodData Central, 2019. fdc.nal.usda.gov

Vona, R., Gambardella, L., & Straface, E. (2018). Gender-associated biomarkers in metabolic syndrome. *Carotid Artery—Gender and Health [Working Title].* https://doi.org/10.5772/intechopen.81103

WebMD. (2020, October 26). *Foods high in MSG.* WebMD. https://www.webmd.com/diet/foods-high-in-msg

Williams, C. (2021, January 26). *Top 5 benefits of meal planning, according to an expert.* Cooking Light. https://www.cookinglight.com/eating-smart/smart-choices/meal-planning-benefits

Image References

Note: All images not included in this reference listing are copyright of the author.

Castorly Stock. (2020). *Cooking utensil on close up*. Pexels. https://www.pexels.com/photo/cooking-utensil-on-close-up-photography-3682218/

Guiraldelli, R. (2021, August 15). *A stainless oven temperature gauge*. Pexels. https://www.pexels.com/photo/a-stainless-oven-thermometer-gauge-9182633/

Husko, V. (2021). *Lemon garlic shrimp*. Pexels, https://www.pexels.com/photo/shrimp-dish-with-sliced-lemon-and-dill-garnish-8633745/

Kobruseva, O. (2020). *Chicken meat on ceramic plate*. Pexels. https://www.pexels.com/photo/chicken-meat-on-white-ceramic-plate-5769384/

Lukas. (2018, March 22). *Sliced vegetables*. Pexels. https://www.pexels.com/photo/sliced-vegetables-952479/

May, C. (2020, November 8), *Kitchen room with white wall*. Pexels. https://www.pexels.com/photo/kitchen-room-with-white-wall-5824883/

Olsson, E. (2018, November 29). *Three trays of food*. Pexels. https://www.pexels.com/photo/flat-lay-photography-of-three-tray-of-foods-1640775/

Olsson, E. (2018b). *Three mason jars inlined on white surface*. Pexels. https://www.pexels.com/photo/three-mason-jars-inlined-on-white-surface-1640776/

Raic, V. (2015). *Scale diet fat health*. Pixabay. https://pixabay.com/photos/scale-diet-fat-health-tape-weight-403585/